VortexHealing®

DIVINE ENERGY HEALING

A Magical Path

of Healing & Awakening

Ric A. Weinman

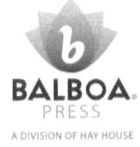

BALBOA.
PRESS
A DIVISION OF HAY HOUSE

Balboa Press books may be ordered through booksellers or by contacting:

Balboa Press
A Division of Hay House
1663 Liberty Drive
Bloomington, IN 47403
www.balboapress.com
1 (877) 407-4847

Because of the dynamic nature of the Internet, any web addresses or links contained in this book may have changed since publication and may no longer be valid. The views expressed in this work are solely those of the author and do not necessarily reflect the views of the publisher, and the publisher hereby disclaims any responsibility for them.

The author of this book does not dispense medical advice or prescribe the use of any technique as a form of treatment for physical, emotional, or medical problems without the advice of a physician, either directly or indirectly. The intent of the author is only to offer information of a general nature to help you in your quest for emotional and spiritual well-being. In the event you use any of the information in this book for yourself, which is your constitutional right, the author and the publisher assume no responsibility for your actions.

VortexHealing® Divine Energy Healing is a complementary energetic healing tool. It is not a replacement for medical treatment. Please consult your physician for medical issues in addition to any complementary healing you receive.

Any people depicted in stock imagery provided by Thinkstock are models, and such images are being used for illustrative purposes only. Certain stock imagery © Thinkstock.

Print information available on the last page.

ISBN: 978-1-5043-3023-7 (sc)
ISBN: 978-1-5043-3024-4 (e)

Library of Congress Control Number: 2015904698

Balboa Press rev. date: 5/27/2015

VortexHealing®

is a holistic system of energetic healing

that works solely with divine light and consciousness,

to heal, to transform,

and to awaken freedom within the human heart.

Dedicated to Merlin,

my divine benefactor.

What a blessing

to have received such Grace.

Acknowledgements

I want to thank my wife, Susanne, and fellow VortexHealing® teacher, Anthony Gorman, for their insights and feedback on the manuscript. I especially want to thank fellow VortexHealing® teacher, Lorraine Goldbloom. People have been asking me to write this book for years, but Lorraine's strong sense that it needed to be written now had enough divine force behind it that all I could do was surrender and write it. In addition, her commitment to this project through her continuous and ongoing support and feedback, at every step along the way, has made a huge impact on the final version of the book you are reading today.

I also want to thank the various VortexHealing® students who shared their healing and awakening stories here, as those stories bring heart and real livingness to the text of the book.

A Note from the Author...

This book is an exploration of an extraordinary healing art
that has become inseparable from the rest of my life.
I am the founder of VortexHealing® Divine Energy Healing,
or more precisely, the *re*-founder, since VortexHealing is
actually an ancient healing art that was lost long ago.

I am also the current lineage holder of this divine lineage.
However, this book isn't about my own journey;
it is about the amazing gift I received
and have been blessed to be able to teach others.

Contents

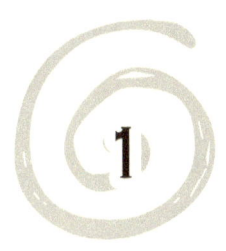

1 VortexHealing® Divine Energy Healing

VortexHealing is a divine gift for healing and awakening. When I first received this, in a rather wild, transcendent kind of experience, I thought it was simply an amazing new healing tool for me to use for my own self-healing and in my full-time healing practice. However, this egocentric idea was entirely wrong: I was there to birth it out into the world, to teach it, and to facilitate its growth and evolution. Although I began by using it for myself and my clients, that was just the starting point.

From the moment VortexHealing came into my life, it took on a life of its own. Its power and effectiveness quickly started to draw attention to itself, and soon there were many requests for me to teach it. Eventually I did, and before long I had to give up my personal healing practice, because I was teaching VortexHealing full-time, in many areas of the world. Starting with its first class, taught in Tucson, in 1995, it has grown into the various levels of classes it is today, taught worldwide by a dedicated group of certified teachers. It has evolved into not just an extraordinary healing art but also a modern-era path for spiritual awakening. I can't begin to express how blessed I feel to be part of this.

The magic of VortexHealing is best experienced first-hand to truly sense both its depth and its grace. Yet the closest we can come to that here is through the sharing of personal experiences. So, in lieu of being able to offer you a direct experience, I present lots of first-hand stories throughout the book, both my own and those of our students.

As you'll see, VortexHealing is quite unique. To really understand what it is and does, one has to look at the world through its eyes. So I'll start by sharing its own bigger picture.

Healing and Awakening

VortexHealing's point of view is that all of life is One (One Source, One Consciousness, One Divinity), expressing Itself as an amazing experience of creation. Yet because we have lost the awareness of that, our basic experience of life has become focused through the narrow lens of separation. We experience ourselves as a particular being, separate from everything else in creation and separate from the Universal Source of creation. This creates all kinds of issues and false identities, which over time (and lives) imprint and condition every level of our human system— our bodies, our minds, our emotions, and even our sense of spirituality. The web of this conditioning is incredibly, almost unimaginably deep. It exists on multi-dimensional levels, and it completely distorts our experience of being human. In addition to creating a myriad of emotional issues, it also creates blockages in our human energy system, which generate weakness and physical disease. All of this traps us in struggle and suffering. We get angry, we get anxious, we feel victimized, we feel lonely, we feel insecure, and/or we become overwhelmed by loss, by our job, or by our family. All of these experiences condition us in a way that strengthens our identity with these places, trapping us even more deeply within them, and deepening our experience of separateness. The intent of VortexHealing is to release this conditioning on every level where it is found, returning the person to emotional balance and energetic strength so that health and happiness prevail.

However, the goal of VortexHealing is also much larger than this, because deeper healing requires a return to wholeness. Wholeness requires a return to the awareness of what we are, an awakening out of our root experience of separation and suffering into the experience of inner freedom that is at the heart of our being. So the divine Source of VortexHealing designed a system of healing to facilitate this kind of awakening. As a result, whether studying or receiving VortexHealing, a process is engaged—a kind of spiritual acceleration process—in which participants begin to awaken out of their conditioned, multi-dimensional webs of reality and identity. Although the healing tools of VortexHealing are designed to generate physical and emotional transformation (and I hope to demonstrate that they do so fantastically), on a deeper level they also engage a process with Divinity that facilitates the deepest movement of healing possible: an inner awakening to the freedom and oneness that is our true nature.

Healing Specific Conditions

We tend to think of healing as a process that gets us well when we have a disease in our physical body. Because we live in a Western industrial culture, we tend to separate what is happening in our body from what is happening to us mentally, emotionally, and spiritually. Of course, there are a variety of situations in which this is true. For instance, someone is caught out in the rain, gets pneumonia, and takes an antibiotic that heals their disease. In this situation, we would say that the drug healed the pneumonia. But this kind of healing-by-drug applies to just a small percentage of issues for which we seek healing.

Consider how this simple example changes if the person is actually quite prone to lung infections. Now there is a chronic situation, but the drug has only treated the acute manifestation. Although the drug manages to clear the latest infection, it has not created true healing. True healing requires treating the pre-existing, chronic condition.

There are many reasons why a person may become prone to lung infections, but most will fall into one of two general categories: either the person has a constitutional weakness or there is an emotional basis that has weakened the body and its energy system in specific ways, making it more susceptible to disease. If the situation is due to constitutional weakness, then a healing modality that can treat constitutional weakness is needed. If the situation has an emotional root, then what is needed is a healing modality that can treat both the emotional basis and the way this has weakened the body's energy system. So to create good physical health, one would ideally use a healing modality such as VortexHealing that can treat both weak constitutional energy and underlying emotional issues.

Of course, physical disease is not the only thing people seek healing for. In the days when I had a healing practice (before I was teaching full-time), most of my clients sought healing to 'feel better'. They didn't have specific illnesses, but they weren't as happy or content as they knew they could be. Some of them were simply seeking relief from obvious, in-their-face emotional issues, such as anger, sadness, rejection, etc. Some of them were simply seeking a weekly energy 'tune-up', only to discover that a big part of what was throwing them out of harmony were background emotional issues that were not being addressed.

Healing our emotional issues, though, is not such an easy thing. Like an iceberg, only the surface of the issue is visible. The rest of the issue lurks in deeper parts of the psyche, supported by both conscious and unconscious identities, supported by past-life memory and ancestral history carried in the DNA. All of this is held on multi-dimensional levels and has conditioned the body (also a multi-dimensional structure) to change in ways to help hold the issue in place. The issue will be imprinted into every aspect of the body's energy system. This cannot be healed without the whole of it being transformed.

That process involves working on all levels of the consciousness of the issue, as well as working with the complex patterns of the body's energy system. For this, we have developed multi-dimensional maps of the psyche and the body's energy system. The maps enable us to work *comprehensively*: on the deepest roots of an issue, on all the other areas of the psyche that support the issue, and on all the levels of the issue in the body's energy system.

Yet there is a deeper level here. In addition to what is held in the body and the psyche, the core of every emotional issue is rooted in our basic experience of separation. Ultimately, that separateness needs to be transformed—by awakening it. However, for a healing modality to accomplish this, it must access a level of energy and consciousness that is already awake and free of separateness, with the power to penetrate to the root of the iceberg. It needs Divinity. Nothing else has the depth or power to do this.

This is why VortexHealing works solely with divine energy and consciousness. This is why it is not just a healing art but also an awakening path: the same divine power that is available for healing the separateness within one's issues can be used for even deeper healing—the awakening of separateness in the core of one's being. People often come to the idea of spiritual awakening through an emotional process of working on specific issues. At some point, they realize that there is a deeper kind of disturbance in their psyche, a certain kind of emptiness in their heart that is at the root of all their suffering. This leads them to seek something more. They become seekers of true spiritual awakening, and some of them find their way to the Divinity within VortexHealing for that, for awakening in this lifetime.

When we do healing on an emotional issue or an injury, this is our context. We are not simply fixing something that is stuck or broken; we are bringing the being back to wholeness, supporting their process of awakening to what they truly are.

VortexHealing® and Divine Expressions

Our universe is rooted in mystery. Something came into being where before there was nothing. How that happens is pure mystery. We also call this "magic". Not the illusionary magic of stage magicians or mentalists, of course, but true magic, which is the power of Divinity to manifest its own potentiality. This is the magic that brings creation into being, that can create miracles, and that you once believed in as a child. This is the magic that touches your heart and helps you to remember who you really are. VortexHealing is about this kind of magic—true magic, from the heart of Divinity, used for healing and inner transformation.

Divinity is completely transcendent—beyond all knowing and being. However, Divinity is capable of creating pure divine expressions out of Itself that can be manifested within creation. The idea of the Holy Trinity in Christianity embodies this concept: God is one and yet has unique expressions. In Hinduism, the various gods are really the various expressions of the One Unfathomable Reality, often referred to as Brahma. Both Christianity and Hinduism believe that one can relate to these expressions and interact with them as if they were beings. In Hinduism, such divine expressions are called avatars (a word that was co-opted by computer science to mean something very different). If Christians used this terminology, they would call Jesus an avatar, since they consider him the "son of God" and simultaneously not distinct from God. Every avatar expresses and embodies a unique quality of Divinity. VortexHealing was created by the divine expression that embodies the quality of transformational magic.

An important aspect of this divine, transformational magic is love. Divine love. (This connection between love and magic is often found in the lyrics of love songs.) Love is completely transformational, and it is the aspect of divinity that human consciousness most easily recognizes and responds to. VortexHealing bridges in this magical quality of divine love in a palpable way in all its healings.

VortexHealing is much more than a healing art. It is a complete transformational process, empowered by Divinity to work with this transformational magic and its expression as love. It brings divine energy and consciousness to anything in creation that needs it. In practice, this enables VortexHealing to work in a very powerful way on the body, the mind, the emotions, and the spiritual consciousness. It impacts all aspects of the body's energy system and transforms the deepest karmic issues we hold as human beings. Because what is being used is always sourced from divine energy and consciousness, the result is not just relaxation or the release of conditioning but the transformation and evolution of human consciousness, awakening it to its true nature.

The VortexHealing® Lineage is the Merlin Lineage

VortexHealing was re-discovered in 1994, but it is part of a lineage that has been on Earth for over 2700 years. (A lineage occurs when a specific teaching is passed down through the generations.) The healing and transformational teachings of VortexHealing lineage are empowered by the divine avataric 'being' that brought it into existence. That avatar, that divine expression, refers to itself as "Merlin". This is not the human being named Merlin associated with King Arthur. That Merlin was one of the teachers of this lineage. Historically, if a VortexHealing teacher reached a certain level of oneness with the divine Source of the lineage, they took on the name Merlin as a title. I am the 13th Merlin in this lineage, and all the VortexHealing teachers living at this time hold this title.

The divine Source of this lineage is the original Merlin. Merlin-0, if you will. It is not coincidental that the name Merlin has always been associated with magic, because that is the nature of this lineage. It is a magical lineage, powered by Divinity, through an avatar that refers to itself as "Merlin". This is Divinity expressing itself as magical transformation. This is the Merlin lineage.

Most spiritual practices have spiritual evolution or awakening as their sole focus. Most healing practices have the teaching of healing as their sole focus. The Merlin lineage has always focused on both. Yet because of the tremendous power in this lineage, it also has other responsibilities. In addition to its focus on spiritual evolution and healing, it has always taken on a certain responsibility for the state of the planet as a whole, doing global healing, both for issues within humanity in general and for individual global conflicts. That kind of work is still done today by both the teachers and the students of the lineage. In fact, one of the healing tools taught in the second level class is specific for doing this kind of work. We use divine magic for global evolution.

In ancient times, Merlin manifested a huge 'divine package' of his energy and consciousness on Earth, with the intention for that package to be the foundation of the Merlin lineage here. In recent times, more of that package has been activated, enabling the Merlin lineage to evolve considerably from what it was in ancient times. The healing tools and the ability to facilitate spiritual awakening keep deepening and are a quantum jump from what they originally were. This is aligned with the acceleration of humanity as a whole: Merlin is making more power available to support this acceleration, facilitating transformation on all levels, both individually and in the larger group field.

Channeling VortexHealing®

VortexHealing is manifested by 'channeling' it either to oneself or someone else. This kind of channeling has nothing to do with trances or trance-like states. VortexHealers are fully conscious and in a normal state of mind, and are simply being a vehicle for divine energies and consciousness to pass through them for the sake of healing. Many energy-healing modalities channel some kind of energy. What makes VortexHealing unique and powerful is not the act of channeling but *what* we channel, *how deeply* into the receiver's system we channel it, and the fact that the channeling is guided by divine intelligence.

In addition, this inner guidance enables the VortexHealer to simply intend to accomplish a particular task with the healing energy, and the divine intelligence within VortexHealing directs the healing to wherever it needs to go to facilitate that. Deep things can happen without the healer having any psychic ability whatsoever.

Why Would Someone Learn VortexHealing®?

People come to VortexHealing for a variety of reasons. Regardless of the reason they start with, though, in one way or another it changes their life. Even if someone just takes the Basic/Foundational class, their energy system goes through a tremendous light-acceleration; they thin out their incarnational drama, they learn to meditate and dialogue with Divinity, and they learn an amazing energetic healing art that they can use on themselves or others, for physical or emotional issues.

For many, that is just the beginning. Some come to VortexHealing because they have seen what this has done, long-term, for their friends. They see how their friends, using VortexHealing, have transformed both emotionally and physically, becoming more centered, more grounded, and more whole. They see that these friends have grown into a deeper sense of inner freedom. Their friends have become less reactive to situations and have more inner space in which to enjoy life. There is a different level of light in their eyes.

Other people become interested in VortexHealing because they have become aware that it is a direct path to spiritual awakening and they want to experience that in this life.

Some people consciously sense the amount of Grace that is available to them in this lineage, and they take the class because they want that to be a part of their lives. And there are those who just want an opportunity to play with the magical divine energy that becomes available to them in VortexHealing.

Interestingly, most new students say they didn't have a conscious reason for taking the class, but when they first heard about VortexHealing, something within them lit up and resonated, and they knew they needed to come. Any specifics they could sense were unconscious, but the call was strong enough to bring them to class.

Regardless of why people come to VortexHealing, that divine Grace is there for everyone. And it transforms their lives.

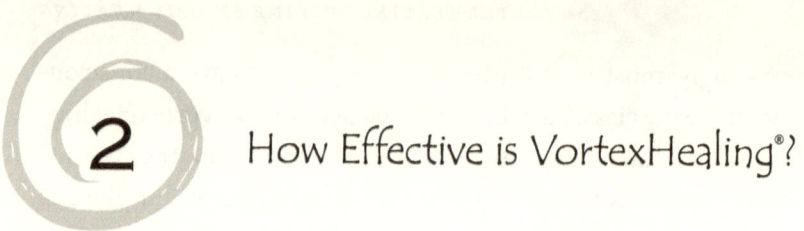

2 How Effective is VortexHealing®?

The first chapter of this book presented you with an overview of VortexHealing. It described the accessing of divine energy and consciousness for healing, and how this kind of healing is also a process for awakening. It is easy to create an appealing philosophy for a healing modality, but how transformative is VortexHealing in actuality? All the descriptions about how divine intention is facilitating healing and transformation will count for nothing if, at the end of the day, VortexHealing just isn't that powerful. This is really the bottom line: How effective is VortexHealing?

Transforming Illness

My first healing experience with VortexHealing: I had been practicing energy healing for about 20 years when, in a wild, peak experience in 1994, I recovered VortexHealing. (See *Chapter 9: History of the VortexHealing® Lineage*, for a description of that initial experience.) At the time, I had been working with Jin Shin Jyutsu®, craniosacral therapy, visceral release (organ massage), unwinding the fascia, and the kind of aura balancing taught in my first book, *Your Hands Can Heal*. I was also fairly psychic, which enabled me to work directly with consciousness as well as see what was working and how well it worked.

One of the first clients to come in after I first recovered VortexHealing had been suffering from chronic fatigue syndrome for about 20 years. To deal with it, he had been practicing Jin Shin Jyutsu® for most of that time. The Jin Shin had softened his symptoms but had never actually cured him of the illness. When I used my psychic sensing to 'look into his body', I saw the chronic fatigue as a virus in his lymph system. (Viral chronic fatigue, to my perception, can be caused by a virus in the lymph system, in one or both kidneys, or a combination of these. As the man got off the healing table, he felt that something had fundamentally changed in his system. This is what he told me afterwards:

> I had chronic fatigue for 20 years. Sometimes it was worse than others. When it was bad I could only be on my feet four hours a day. I could get groceries and do some errands, and then I'd have to rest. When it was better I could walk around for six hours a day. I got involved with alternative healing methods because there was nothing doctors could do. But I couldn't get rid of it. Then, after more than 20 years, I met you and you used VortexHealing on me. I was lying on my stomach, and you put your hands over my kidneys. When I sat up again, I felt like I had been in deep meditation; I had a peaceful, soothing feeling. After those three days I noticed my energy level coming up again. I knew the chronic fatigue was gone. And it has stayed gone. Just from that one session.

I have encountered many of these kinds of cases over the years, and unless there are other mitigating factors, most of these long-term, viral-based chronic fatigue situations tend to be shifted with VortexHealing in one to three sessions.

Experiences in India: Soon after the above healing, I went to India for a couple of weeks to sit with a spiritual teacher named H.W.L. Poonja, also simply called Papaji. While there, I was allowed to do some energy healing sessions on Papaji, and I was invited to eat with him. Usually he ate in silence, but occasionally he would suddenly start talking about someone in the community who was ill with one condition or another. I interpreted that as him pointing me to do healing on them, which I was happy to do. Here are a couple of those stories:

> The first person Papaji pointed me to had acute leukemia and was under medical care, getting regular blood transfusions. To my perception, he had a virus in his bone marrow. His body was trying to knock the virus out with white blood cells,

but because it wasn't able to accomplish this, it just kept producing more and more of them. This over-production of white blood cells was perceived by Western medicine as the disease, but to my perception, the disease was the virus in the bone marrow. I did three VortexHealing treatments on him, and I heard later that over the next month all of his blood indicators for the leukemia had cleared up.

My sense is that most autoimmune diseases involve a virus. For instance, my perception of Multiple Sclerosis is that a virus has gotten into the nerves. In attempting to kill the virus, the immune system attacks the nerves, which creates more damage than the virus itself.

Here is another story from my time with Papaji, in which a virus was generating chronic illness:

One of Papaji's helpers had gotten very ill. On a trip with Papaji, she had developed two simultaneous cases of hepatitis. She was flat on her back with no energy, and she was told she would be like this for the rest of her life. I could see two large 'swirls' in her liver that gave off the kind of energetic frequency that viruses give off. I had never seen viral swirls in a liver before. I did four VortexHealing sessions with her, and towards the end of the last session, both of the viral swirls, to my perception, disappeared. When that happened, the woman felt her energy come flooding back into her body, and when the session was over she was back on her feet and felt fine. I saw her some days later, and the healing had held; her energy was back to normal.

Shifting the Genetics: The genetic system is extremely hard to access with healing energy. Unfortunately, there are healing modalities that falsely believe they are changing the code of the DNA, and some of their language indicates they have no understanding of what science actually knows about our genetics. This gives alternative healing a reputation as being unscientific and operating from fantasy. When the genetics change, the physiology changes, and this can be measured in laboratory testing. VortexHealing cannot change the structure of DNA, but we do seem to be able to affect genetic *expression*. Here is a story about this, regarding my own body:

> *At the time VortexHealing came into my life, I had what is called Gilbert's Syndrome, a genetic liver condition that causes bilirubin, a liver enzyme, to be improperly processed. It is not a harmful condition, but in blood tests, the bilirubin readings will be high. Mine were sky high. When VortexHealing developed the ability to impact genetic expression, I did what we call a "genetic modification" on myself for the Gilbert's Syndrome, and a couple of months later when I had my blood re-tested, my bilirubin levels had dropped so far they were now within normal range. Since Gilbert's is diagnosed by high bilirubin readings, a blood test would no longer diagnose that for me.*

Being able to impact the genetics can obviously play an important role for certain kinds of disease situations. As we'll see later, all the ancestral memory that is carried in the DNA—which is emotional memory—impacts not just the body but also generates and supports various emotional issues. Being able to access this level is especially critical for dealing with emotional patterns of struggle and survival.

Weak Constitutional Energy: Many people get ill simply because they have a weak 'constitution'. Even an untrained eye observing a room full of children can pick out one or two who look like they will easily get ill. It's clear they are missing some kind of core strength and basic vitality that is visible in the other children. Over the years I have observed that a good percentage of adults with chronic disease patterns started life with a weak constitution. More specifically, they began life with a low level of at least one constitutional energy, most commonly the kidney energy. That percentage approaches 100% for certain illnesses, such as MS (Multiple Sclerosis). The weak kidney energy makes the system susceptible to the kinds of viruses that can create autoimmune situations. Here is an example:

I noticed during a class that one of the students was dragging her leg when she walked. Turned out she had MS, and when I checked her system I could sense a virus in her nervous system. Knocking out the virus didn't take very long, and within a few days she was walking normally. I had her work on her constitutional kidney energy, which was weak, and she has not had a relapse since.

Unfortunately, constitutional energy never gets stronger by itself without some kind of energetic intervention. Most healing modalities will make the system seem stronger but won't get to the constitutional level. As a result, if treatment is not maintained, the system will become weak again. With the more advanced VortexHealing tools, we can strengthen the constitutional energy, so we check that for weakness when we are dealing with chronic illness, and strengthen it if we find any.

The Larger Picture with Illness: Although many illnesses can be addressed by simply paying attention to the physical body and its energy system, most chronic illness will also have emotional issues as an important component. Diseases such as cancer, in addition to genetic tendencies and environmental factors, will typically have an emotional component at its root. Even when an illness starts out as purely a physical condition, when the illness sits in the body over a period of time, it will bring up emotions such as helplessness, anger, or grief, and these not only become part of the disease pattern but act to hold it in place.

Transforming Other Body Conditions

Not all body conditions are illnesses. Burns, injuries, low energy, weakness, back pain, and so on, are examples of such body conditions.

In *Chapter 5: Student Healing Stories,* you'll read many examples of healing these kinds of non-illness conditions from students' own experiences. Here is a quick story, shared by a student, to illustrate how effective VortexHealing can be:

I treated a woman who had a burn to her arm that had become so infected it had created a deep festering hole that needed to be packed weekly. She had had it for months and been treated with antibiotics etc. She was awaiting surgery to have it cut away and have skin grafted. I did one treatment. It healed completely within four days. The nurse who had been packing it said it was a miracle.

Transforming Emotional Issues

Our emotional issues are the places where we feel stuck or get caught emotionally. They are the places where we have fixed emotional reactions to life situations. If you feel insecure at work because your boss doesn't tell you how well you are doing, that is an emotional issue. If you are chronically depressed or irritated, those are emotional issues. If you have chronic anxiety, or loneliness, or hopelessness, whether in general or only in relation to certain situations, these are all emotional issues. An emotional issue is any fixed reaction pattern that we have to life situations. Typically, though, we only own them as issues when they get triggered on a regular basis.

If you have worked on trying to clear up an emotional issue and change your reactivity, you know how stubborn these issues can be.

The Difficulty with Emotional Issues: It would seem that it should be easy to change what arises in us emotionally. But emotional issues are very comprehensive. The fact that they can so fully take us over, in spite of all our efforts to heal or avoid them, shows how comprehensive they are. All emotional issues are body *and* mind issues. Some aspects of the issue will be held in our psyche and some aspects will be held as conditioning in the body. At the core of every issue is an identity, which means that you experience that emotional state as what you are. The identity will be supported by eons of history, and it will have genetic (ancestral memory) support and a lifetime of lived history. All of this generates conditioning for the issue that permeates every aspect of our body's energy system. Below, and in *Chapter 6: The Human Package,* you will find a fuller description of how we hold an issue in these places. The details do not tell the whole story, but they create a good outline of what we are dealing with when we address issues.

Issues Held in the Psyche: When we say that an issue is held in our psyche, we also mean our mind or consciousness. The assumption is typically that it is held in a single spot in consciousness. But the consciousness of it exists on many levels and in many different 'rooms' of our psyche. Generally speaking, the issue will be held in three main areas of consciousness: the incarnational consciousness (past-life memory), the genetic consciousness, and the consciousness of the human personality. Its expression in these places include the emotion of the issue, the historical memories of the issue (including past lives, present life, and genetic/ancestral memories), our identities with the issue, and a complete mental mind-set full of attitudes and beliefs. All of these are part of the complex of the issue. It is important to understand that the consciousness of an issue cannot be dealt with simply by trying to re-program a belief. The whole complex needs to be transformed.

Therapy can help shift some of the consciousness of an issue, but in therapy we mostly access the conscious personality. The roots of issues are deeper, held in deeper layers of the psyche. The beauty of VortexHealing is that its divine intelligence takes it to wherever it needs to go to transform the issue.

A student who had only taken the Basic/Foundational training shared a story with me about a woman she had treated:

> She told me that the woman—we'll call her M—was living at home with her mother and brother. She was brought in by her mother. M was extremely depressed and destructive. Sometimes she would cut up the electric cables in her house. She had not eaten for days, and the mother described her as, "behaving like someone possessed." She even arrived in her pajamas because she refused to get dressed, and she wasn't too happy about being there. The student said, "There was such a sense of sadness about her, but I told her that 'we would laugh together yet'." The student did four sessions. She

said that about an hour before M arrived for the last session,
she got a very deep sense of M and knew that her healing had
taken place. She said, "M arrived all smiles. At one point, we
laughed and laughed." M was then able to go back to work.
She got a job in the kitchen of a very busy pub.

It is hard to know exactly what Merlin transformed within this woman to create the healing, but some aspect of her *identity* with the depression would have needed to be part of that. To have an identity with something means that in some way you use it to access your experience of self. So when we are angry we say, "I am angry." When we are depressed we say, "I am depressed." There is no separation between the experience of what you are and the anger or depression. You are using those emotions as a way of accessing a sense of self. You believe in the validity of the identity, and more beliefs will come into being to support that position until there is a whole mind-set supporting it. Once established, there will always be sufficient material in the form of present and past-life experiences to support any emotional identity that you presently hold, even if that identity was created in a past life.

An experience I had treating a dyslexic woman points to how identity can even influence our perceptual system:

I did a few very short sessions (10-15 minutes each) on
a woman who was a severe dyslexic. The woman was a
professional cook, but her condition was so bad that not
only couldn't she read properly, she could hardly read her
own labels that she put on food containers. The cause of her
condition seemed to be a strong emotional identity with a
non-human body and perceptual system she had experienced
in a past life. In that life, her perceptual system was very
non-linear. Her identity kept her in that non-linear state and
made the simple act of reading a food label very difficult. Soon
after the 3rd session, I came across her reading a magazine,
which would have been impossible earlier. In addition, her
manager told me that she now interacted in a different way,

because she could "stack ideas in her mind now", allowing
her to have more complex conversations.

An identity can be rooted in either our incarnational consciousness (including our lives on other planets) or in our genetic/ancestral consciousness. It can arise out of either thread of lived history, but because of the way these two areas of consciousness interact, every identity will show up in both places. For a healing art to clear the issue, therefore, it must be able to work effectively in both the incarnational and genetic consciousness.

Issues Rooted in Separation: Identity is the key to an issue, but identity has its own deeper root. We find that root by asking: Why do we create identities to define ourselves? It's because we are operating from a sense of self that is separate. We believe that our sense of personal, separate 'I' and 'me' is who we really are. Yet because this is ultimately untrue, there is an inherent insecurity in our experience of self. So we try to protect ourselves. We create identities to bolster our existence, to solidify our sense of self against the insecurity we feel inside. However, no matter how much we add to a lie, it is still a lie, and lies have consequences. When we lie to ourselves about who we are, the consequences are the identities we create to support the lie, which generate the issues and drama that trap us in suffering.

Exploring this dynamic deeper, our inherent insecurity also creates a basic sense of lack and a loss of true safety. This drives us into survival consciousness. We feel threatened and that we need to struggle to survive. Although we push this awareness into the background to avoid feeling the suffering it creates, in one way or another, we end up projecting this inner drama onto almost everything going on in our lives.

Instead of being open and spontaneous, we develop fixed reaction patterns to life situations. Our lives become a constant compensation for our inner drama and become oriented around filling our sense of lack and creating a sense of safety. But whatever we do is never enough—and it can't be, because a false sense of self can never be whole or safe. It becomes like quicksand, where the more we struggle, the deeper we go, and our suffering becomes more acute, even if we push the knowing of that to the background.

Inside, we feel the loss of freedom. Yet ironically, because we developed all this identity and inner drama as a means of self-protection, we are also attached to it in spite of the suffering it creates. We still believe—regardless of the fact that it hasn't worked—that the solution is to continue to bolster our sense of separate self.

This story shows what can happen when a key piece of the sense of separate self is released, illustrating its role as the underlying foundation for all our identities and issues. The story is a student's experience after her first movement of awakening:

> *It's like my whole life was always lived from 'within' issues, conditioning, emotions etc., and I was constantly in a state of reacting to them and/or trying to control my reactions— which means my life was always being created from a reaction to an issue, conditioning, or emotion. Now it is not. Issues are still happening and it is not always smooth, but this is an entirely different existence. Whatever 'I am', it is not issues or conditioning or emotions. Big BIG liberation.*

Issues Held in the Body & Energy System: Although we think of issues as being in our psyche, all issues will express through the body, and the resulting tension patterns, which tend to become permanent due to body memory, help to hold the issue in place. Issues are typically held almost *everywhere* in the body, with a stronger focus in one or several areas. Think of what happens when you get angry: everything in your body tightens into a particular overall body position, so every cell of your body and every body system, including your brain, gets engaged with that emotion and holds it as memory. This happens within your energy pathways, your chakras, and other aspects of your energy system as well. All of this body memory helps to keeps the issue active in the psyche, so it becomes part of the structure of the issue. There are healing modalities that just focus on reprogramming the brain, but this is only one aspect of what is held of an issue in the body. As I wrote earlier, the whole complex of the issue needs to be transformed.

When you read the VortexHealing stories throughout this book, keep in mind that although a particular emotional shift or a particular physical healing may be described in a story, VortexHealing is always working on all the levels it can access—body and mind, energy system and consciousness, beliefs and identity—to create that shift.

This story illustrates how the energy system can impact the psyche:

This happened on one of my trips to India to see Papaji. There was a woman who kept inviting me over to her house to have dinner with her and her boyfriend. I knew that she was more interested in having me do some healing on her boyfriend than she was in feeding me, but I accepted anyway. (By then, with just the few healings I had done on people in the community, I had developed a reputation.) I did some healing on the boyfriend before dinner. I could see that his liver was still in pretty bad shape from hepatitis he had had over ten years ago—it was still pretty yellow to my perception, even though his skin was a normal color. But after putting my hands on his liver and doing VortexHealing for a few minutes, the energy stopped and I knew it was done. The energy had its own intelligence, which I trusted. The couple must have been expecting a much longer session, so they were quite disappointed that I channeled for such a short time, but to their credit, they fed me anyway. I told them that his liver was much better now—I could see that it was—but they were quite doubtful. After all, I had only worked on him for three or four minutes.

The next day, at Papaji's satsang, the woman came running up to me all excited. "He's a new man," she kept saying. "It's as if he was beamed up to a spaceship in the middle of the night by aliens who took out the old personality and replaced it with a new one." She liked the new one much better and would be quite happy if they just kept the old one.

She said he woke up with energy for the first time in as long as she could remember, and he was sweet and helped her with the dishes. He had always been tired and cranky.

I could have spent many hours treating this man's crankiness. However, in this case, more of it was being manifested from his body and energy system than from his psyche. When his liver and liver pathways were restored to harmony, his emotional state shifted as well.

Some issues will need more healing on the level of the body and energy system; some will need more healing in the consciousness. Yet both need to be addressed, for the body and mind are intimately linked. Here is a story that illustrates just how profound that link is:

A man came for a session who had cancer. From a holistic healing perspective, many diseases have an emotional root. The core emotion for cancer is suppressed grief and self-pity. That in turn is fed by resentment and/or hate, which produce a certain kind of acid-toxin in the system that makes it easier for the cancer to grow. This man was obviously self-fermenting in some kind of grief, and definitely feeling self-pity for himself. So I asked him about what was going on for him. It turned out that his best friend had slept with his wife. The resentment poured out of him as he told me about it. And what he kept saying over and over again was, "He stabbed me in the back." There was the connection between his emotions and the disease that was growing in his body, for his cancer was in his back, right where he was feeling and expressing the emotional charge.

I suggested to the man that a key for him in clearing his cancer would be forgiving his friend. In fact, he might have to choose between dying of cancer and forgiving his friend. I only saw him that one time, though, so I don't know what happened to him.

Transforming issues is difficult and multi-faceted. They are very comprehensive and run very deep. In the above descriptions, I don't go into the multi-dimensional levels of our issues, as that would get too technical, but in practice our issues do need to be addressed on all levels, both in the psyche and energy system. You need to get to the deepest roots of the issue and then deal with its conditioning at all levels of consciousness and in the entirety of the body's energy system. All of this makes an issue very difficult to transform. The magic of VortexHealing is that it works on the issue everywhere we hold it, including our identities at the root of the issue, and even the root sense of separateness behind all our identities.

VortexHealing wants to help you get free of your issues, and in the process—as part of that process—it also wants to free you from your sense of separateness, to open you to the vastness of inner freedom.

Transforming the Quality of Life

Transforming emotional issues and illness have a huge impact on the quality of one's life. Yet the sense of inner freedom brings another, ineffable element to the quality of life that transcends these other factors. This student's story describes the recovery of this other element and how VortexHealing helped him in that process:

> Ever since I was a boy, I knew there was something more to life, something "else" out there that most of the people around me seemed unaware of. I didn't have language for it then, but it was definitely something spiritual and something real. After graduating from college, I spent the next twenty years writing, performing, and directing original work for theatre and film. For me, the creative act was a spiritual activation, as I learned to be wholly present in my body, to identify and express emotions with nonattachment, and to be open to something larger than myself that could write the words, act the speech, and direct the play.
>
> A fairly traumatic event in my life led me to VortexHealing, and the result of that first session was so dramatic and profound that I knew I had to study this healing art for myself. I may not have known it then, but my

physical life and my spiritual search were becoming one, so that now I can no longer distinguish between the two. Instead of experiencing a sense of duality between my physical self here and something spiritual "out there", now there is an undeniable connection between my physical experience of life with a palpable spiritual reality that is here and everywhere simultaneously. This truth is reinforced every time I give a healing session to a client. No matter what is going on for me that day, when I am in the presence of this healing energy it magically transforms the entire experience so that the client and I, and everything and everyone we come in contact with, is changed from that moment on.

I now feel more connected to a deeper version or vision of myself than I ever thought was possible. My life is no longer a haphazard, random series of events with only me and my self-interests at the center, but one in which a larger, more graceful, loving, and intimately alive presence continuously weaves itself through me like a mischievous and kind fabric, never leaving me alone.

Healing at a Distance

With VortexHealing, sessions can be done in person or at a distance, and the distance work is very effective. Healing at a distance is possible because everything is really connected—both in consciousness and in the energetic field that makes up physical reality—and the VortexHealing transmissions facilitate the bridging of healing energy through that connectedness.

Many of the healing stories you'll read in this book were done at a distance, but unless that is mentioned in the story, the session could have been done either way. However, here is an example of distance healing that I did myself. This was actually a series of short healings, each one lasting 15 minutes or less, done on an autistic boy. Over a time span of some six years, I have done about nine of these short sessions on him. This is what his mother wrote recently, summarizing her son's progress:

23

When you first worked with C (when he was 6 years old), he showed improved eye contact. He began to express humor and show some interest in amusing others. In fourth grade, following your working with C, he showed some willingness to interact with others. Before this time he would not sit next to others in school. He began to engage in group activities with other children. In fifth grade, when you worked with him, he began to have some interest in other children and the idea of having friends. C also developed some organizational skills. When you worked with him last year his organizational skills improved further to the point that he no longer needs any special services at school and has been on high honors with distinction. He has developed a few close (and many more casual) friends both at school and at the conservatory. C continues to sit with these children at lunchtime and to text them outside of school. He does not choose to interact with them in person outside of school (I believe mostly because he wants to be able use his time to practice the piano). He has expressed a much greater range of emotions including tears and has better emotional regulation most of the time. C's music teacher and other musicians have commented on the "improved color" in C's playing; his expression of emotion in his playing has deepened greatly. Following your most recent work with C, our house has been more relaxed and pleasant. He is more able to let go of discussions even when he does not get his way, and interactions with his sister and her friends have not ended in tears and disagreements. C has also been initiating pleasant, interesting conversation, which has not been based solely around his interests and desires.

Thank you so much for your work with C. I feel so much more positive and hopeful about his abilities and his life.

Transforming Matter and the Sound of Musical Instruments

One of the unique things about VortexHealing, because of how deeply it can 'bridge' its healing capacities into whatever is being worked on, is its ability to transform the sound of musical instruments. This is commented on in most of the articles written about VortexHealing. (Visit *www.vortexhealing.org/articles.htm* to read these.) The very first time I did a healing on a musical instrument was on a friend's violin. She was a professional violinist and played in an orchestra. This is what she told me:

> I was a little doubtful that you could improve the sound of my violin, but I was amazed at how much clearer and cleaner the sound became. It was richer, too. I didn't tell my orchestra leader anything, though, because he would think I was crazy. But when I used it, he asked me if I had gotten a new violin. He could hear how different the sound was.

As another example, a professional violinist brought the violin he used with his students to a public talk about VortexHealing. This is what he later told me he experienced when he played it again after the short healing:

> As the first notes rang out from the strings I could see the jaws of the audience visibly dropping! The sound was totally transformed. This tiny fiddle was now ringing with the type of resonance I usually only expect from the fine antique (200-300 year old) violins I use for professional performance.

Healing a musical instrument requires a healing modality that can transform the vibrational reality of physical matter. The healings on these instruments took less than a minute. So consider this: If VortexHealing can significantly transform the sound quality of an inanimate object in less than a minute, imagine what it can do to a human body and energy system in a full-hour treatment.

Energy healing skeptics like to say that the results from healings are just placebo effects, but musical instruments cannot generate placebo effects. To demonstrate this more scientifically, at one point I took some musical instruments to a sound lab where a sound engineer performed some 'before and after' tests on them with sound-testing equipment. The results of how the sound produced by the instruments changed can be seen at *www.vortexhealing.org/draco.htm.*

VortexHealing students facilitate amazing healings all over the world. In addition to the stories shared in this chapter, many more are shared later in this book, in *Chapter 5: Student Healing Stories.* There are also lots more stories on the VortexHealing website, at http://vortexhealing.org/stories.htm. If you are interested in trying a VortexHealing session or getting one for a friend, a world-wide list of available VortexHealers can be found by clicking on the Find-A-Healer button on our website.

3 What makes VortexHealing®
So Unique & Powerful

VortexHealing clearly impacts both the human consciousness and human body, and it can transform the vibrational quality of physical matter. How is it able to do that? Many factors are at play, contributing to these magical transformations. The key to all of them is an avatar that is sourcing, powering, and directing the VortexHealing lineage. VortexHealing was not created by a human being. It was created by an avatar, a direct expression of Divinity, and it was created with the intention of manifesting a healing art that would have amazing powers to heal and transform. In short, VortexHealing is able to heal and transform in astounding ways because manifested Divinity, from Grace, has intended that it be able to do this, actively providing divine guidance, which permeates every aspect of this healing art.

Although the VortexHealing teachers come up with many of the particulars for the classes, the essence of what happens in each class is designed and given by Merlin, the divine Source of this lineage, the divine expression of transformational magic.

There isn't space here to go into all of the particulars that make VortexHealing so unique and powerful, but this chapter will explore the most important ones.

Below are 15 key elements that make VortexHealing the magical healing art it is. Any one of these would deeply strengthen the power of an energetic healing art. All of them together create a profound healing art that continually amazes:

1. Channeling Divine Energy and Vital Energy

The energy of creation has a particular quality and vibration. We call this energy *vital* energy, or *life force* energy. It has the quality of aliveness.

In the VortexHealing view, the Divinity it was created from has its own kind of energy, called *divine* energy, and it has a higher vibration and a completely different quality than vital energy. One can think of vital energy as divine energy that has been 'slowed down'. Understanding the difference in these energies is important because they have different functions in healing.

Most energy healing modalities use vital-level energy to energize or balance the body's vital energy system. Four fairly well-known examples of this would be Jin Shin Jyutsu®, polarity, Reiki, and healing modalities that work with "prana", which is the Sanskrit word for "life force energy". One could also include acupuncture, since that works with balancing vital energy, even though it uses needles to accomplish this rather than channeling energy. Using vital energy, these kinds of practices can do a nice job of harmonizing the outer layers of the energy system, which releases stress, promotes health, and engages people in their issues. But they cannot penetrate deeply into the core of the body's energy system where the deeper energetic blockages are held, and they cannot work directly in consciousness. You need a different kind of energy for that. You need an energy with a higher frequency, which is divine energy. Although vital energy is originally divine energy that is 'slowed down' so it can function as the livingness of creation, as healing tools these two energies function very differently.

Divine energy, being at a much higher frequency, can penetrate into any kind of energetic blockage no matter how deep it is. It is much more intense and compressed, so as it penetrates these blockages, it can break them up. It's like the difference between regular sound waves and the kind of sound waves used to break up a kidney stone. Using regular sound waves, talking to a kidney stone, or playing music for it all day will have no impact; but the kind of high-focused sound that is used for this can penetrate the stones and break them up.

However, there are certain kinds of health situations where vital energy, if used properly, can have a better impact than divine energy. The most common of these situations is just general fatigue. Vital energy works a little better than divine energy for this. Consequently, there are a few VortexHealing energies that have been slowed down to vibrate as if they were vital energies, to fill that role where vital energy is more useful. Yet most situations that can be helped by vital energy are more complex: what you typically find is one part of the system calling for vital energy while the rest of the system is calling for divine energy. For instance, perhaps there is a deeper energetic block or emotional issue that is causing the fatigue. The fatigue itself is better remedied with vital energy (although divine energy can do almost as well). However, the deeper cause of the fatigue calls for divine energy; vital energy can't clear that. With VortexHealing, both needs are met simultaneously, as both divine and vital-like energies are channeled, guided to where they need to go by divine intelligence.

2. Energetic Specificity

In VortexHealing, at the level of its Basic/Foundational class (the first class that is the prerequisite for all others), there are 49 different and unique forms of divine Vortex energy, each one designed to create a specific effect. For instance, one form of Vortex energy is full of compressed shakti (charged, divine energy) and is designed to be intensely active so it can energize the system, and so it can move and transform emotional and karmic conditioning. Another form of Vortex energy is designed to stabilize the system when it is exhausted or shaky, another form is just for grounding, and another is specific for inflammation. For general emotional healing, one Vortex energy brings in the quality of divine love, while another brings in divine peace, which is very helpful for fear issues. For infections, there is a Vortex energy that specifically burns out viruses and bacteria. There is a Vortex energy specific for integration, one for relaxing the mind, and as written above, there are Vortex energies that have been 'slowed down' to function as vital energies.

One of my favorite Vortex energies, called Intimate Heart Vortex, bridges in the state of intimacy. This can be used in various ways. One way is simply to help someone be more aware of their issue, because Intimate Heart Vortex will bridge them into it, making them more intimate with it. When channeled in a general way, it will illuminate whatever resists intimacy, making this more conscious. In addition, Intimate Heart

Vortex can be channeled into the core of the person's being, intending for it to bridge the person to Divinity. In this way, it can also be used as a meditation, to help open someone to Divinity.

In addition, 33 of the different Vortex energies are specific for healing different kinds of body tissue. They act as energetic blueprints for the various kinds of tissue, carrying the healthy vibrational qualities for those tissues and bridging them into the cells, teaching the cells of those tissues to resonate with those vibrational qualities.

So each of these 49 forms of Vortex energy has been designed to accomplish something unique in the energy system or consciousness, which enables it to do that better than a single, more general energy. And in every situation, the VortexHealing practitioner has a choice: a single Vortex energy can be chosen and channeled to accomplish a particular task, or all 49 forms of Vortex can be channeled simultaneously. When channeled simultaneously, each of the 49 forms of Vortex is automatically sent by the divine intelligence within the energy to exactly where it needs to go.

Another key aspect of the specificity made possible by VortexHealing is that it can be intended to impact any specific spot, organ, or system, at any level. The energy will then get concentrated there—even when channeled at a distance. For instance, Vortex energy can be directed specifically into the meridian system, which creates an acupuncture-like healing; it can be channeled to a specific organ or injury; it can be focused into specific parts of the brain. In later classes, it can even target the genetics or aspects of our system and consciousness at higher dimensional levels.

The energy system is very complex, and the deeper energetic structures will never be touched without a way of channeling specifically into them. In addition, most of these deeper energetic structures need divine energy; vital energy simply does not penetrate deeply enough to reach them.

This ability to target something specifically is just as important when healing emotional issues. Our emotional issues are not simply vague 'emotional states'; they have a structure, with roots held at deeper dimensional levels of our psyche. There is also the aspect of an issue that is held in our energy system. This can include, for instance, emotional fixations and 'charges' (dense areas of highly charged emotional energy) that have deep, dense centers. Reaching and transforming all this in our psyche and energy system requires both specificity and penetrating power.

One of my favorite things to do when I teach a Basic/Foundational class is to have students channel VortexHealing, but to keep changing what they are intending for it to do. For instance, perhaps they start with energizing their meridian pathways, then they use it to bring in a sense of deep peace, then to clear the energetic blockage in an organ or a chakra, then to clear their emotional body, then to help them feel their third eye, then to ground themselves, then to bring in a sense of divine love, etc. It is almost shocking, the first time this is experienced, to see how the same group of Vortex energies, channeled with different intentions, can do so many different things. And this ability of VortexHealing to do so many different things simply grows and deepens with each class.

One extra perk of VortexHealing's energetic specificity is that it can be a vehicle for exploring one's own body and energy system. For instance, people have often heard about chakras (the energy centers along the spine) but have never experienced them. All they would have to do is channel Vortex energy into a particular chakra and tune into the resulting sensation. Never felt your third eye? If Vortex energy is channeled into it, you will feel exactly where that sits in your system—and feeling it can help you bridge your awareness into it and learn how to use it.

3. Divine Intelligence

The reason that the VortexHealing practitioner can focus so specifically on any emotional pattern or any specific part of the body or its energy system, even when channeled at a distance, is because of the divine intelligence inherent within the VortexHealing system. It is this same divine intelligence that enables the practitioner to channel 49 unique forms of Vortex energy simultaneously and have each one sent to where it needs to go in the receiver's system. The channeler does not know where these energies should go. With emotional issues, the channeler will not necessarily know where the key areas of that issue are sitting in the receiver's system and consciousness. But the divine intelligence that is inseparable from the divine energy being channeled knows, and it directs the energy accordingly.

Even when a person presents a very simple situation, such as fatigue, this kind of divine intelligence is needed to properly treat the person. There are many different modalities that will have a way to energize the person, but what of the cause of the fatigue? If it is emotional and that is not dealt with, the person may leave feeling good but a few hours later the fatigue will return. If there are deep energetic blockages involved, they need to be found and cleared. If the fatigue is due to a weak constitution, then the constitutional energy needs to be built up. The fatigue itself may also have created energetic side effects that need to be cleared— usually with divine energy—or else they will re-create the fatigue. With VortexHealing we can channel to help both the fatigue itself and the *cause* of the fatigue. Divine intelligence will direct the energy and divine consciousness to where it needs to go to help both.

One interesting benefit to working with this divine intelligence is that we can learn to interact with it and get answers to yes/no types of questions. This is extremely useful when trying to understand what is happening with a client, and even more useful for personal guidance. It enables VortexHealing students to access divine inner guidance, for all aspects of their lives.

Another important effect of this divine intelligence is that VortexHealing practitioners automatically follow the first law of medicine: Do No Harm. There are actually many situations in which energetic medicine can do harm. With acupuncture, for instance, where the energy system is being balanced according to the understanding of the practitioner, things can be put out of balance. And if a needle is not inserted correctly, it can cause an injury. (I know personally of several cases of this.) With other energy-channeling healing arts, if the receiver is exhausted and the channeled energy is creating movement that the receiver's system needs to process, it can lead to more exhaustion, which will slow down the healing process. The practitioner needs to know when to stop—and in some cases, needs to know when they shouldn't channel at all. The divine intelligence within VortexHealing regulates this.

There are also energy healing modalities that attempt to "reprogram the nervous system". It's a good concept—and one that VortexHealing uses as well—but without divine intelligence doing the reprogramming, it is done according to a fallible human being's mental understanding of what should be reprogrammed and how it should be done. If the practitioner has been taught that a particular response in the system should, for instance, have a certain strength, then they will try to get all of their clients' bodies to act that way, irrespective of individual differences and irrespective of all the other things in the body that need to change as well. Essentially, the practitioner can *override* what is natural for that particular body according to how they think it should be.

With VortexHealing, we don't have to be concerned with the kinds of issues that can arise from faulty human understanding. When the energy needs to stop, the divine intelligence within the energy stops it. If it shouldn't be channeled at all, then as much as the practitioner may want to channel it, nothing will happen. It will be like opening a faucet but no water comes out. If something is being reprogrammed, then there is no concern about overriding the system, for it is divine intelligence that is doing the reprogramming, according to the specific needs of that person.

4. Channeling Divine Consciousness

Usually, when we think of energy healing modalities, we think in terms of channeling some kind of energy to generate a particular kind of transformation in the system being worked on. With VortexHealing, in addition to the divine and vital-like energies being channeled, there is also the ability to channel divine *consciousness*. Divine energy and divine consciousness are, of course, related. Divine energy will have divine consciousness in the background, and divine consciousness will carry some amount of divine energy. Yet each has unique properties and powers.

To understand how this works, consider that we have an energy system and we have a consciousness. If we have an emotional issue, it will be held in our body, in all kinds of different areas of our energy system, and in our consciousness. Divine energy is best suited to work in our energy system, while divine consciousness is best suited to work on our consciousness. So, when working on an issue, the divine energy energizes and transforms that issue, wherever it is conditioned into the various areas of our energy system, at the same time that divine consciousness works on the consciousness of that issue, transforming it directly.

This is much more powerful than just working with the energy or just working with the consciousness—especially since the two interact. Consciousness conditions the energy system and the energy system reflects its conditioning in consciousness, so whatever isn't cleared in one will spread itself back into the other. Both need to be cleared, and when they are cleared simultaneously there is a synergistic effect: as the consciousness shifts, it becomes easier to clear what is conditioned in the energy system, and as the conditioning in the energy system clears, there is less support for the consciousness of the issue, making that easier to clear.

For emotional issues, and for inner evolution and transformation, the consciousness aspect of the healing, of course, is much more critical than the energetic aspect. Most energy healing modalities have no ability to address the consciousness of an issue; they only work with the energy system. With VortexHealing, though, not only is the consciousness addressed, but it is *pinpointed* by divine intelligence, so the consciousness of the core of the issue—its very identity—is worked on and transformed. The divine intelligence also knows exactly where all the supports for that consciousness sit in the energy system, enabling divine *energy* to specifically address those, at the same time that the emotional core of the issue is being transformed by divine *consciousness*.

5. Divine Magic & Divine Love

In addition to the role that divine consciousness plays in VortexHealing, as described above, that consciousness also has a unique inner quality— the quality of divine, transformational magic and love. This love is not the same as human romantic love. Although human romantic love will have its root in divine love, the experience of it is filtered through the complex egoic lens of personal self and all the baggage that comes with that: lack, desire, neediness, sexuality, fears of intimacy and vulnerability, emotional insecurity, and so on. Human love comes closest to divine love in that first magical moment in which it is experienced, when two hearts touch and open together in innocence, before all the other stuff in the psyche distorts what has happened in that moment. Even then, it remains just a shadow of true divine love, which is unfettered, unfiltered, and the essence of the power behind all creation. When VortexHealing is channeled, the divine consciousness carries this incredible quality of love within its general divine expression as transformational magic. The divine love coming through the healing is quite palpable, and human emotional consciousness responds very powerfully to it, adding more transformational power to what is already happening in the healing.

This deep quality of love is also present in all 49 of the divine Vortex energies, but more in the background with most of them, since each of the Vortex energies has its own specific quality. The love is also quite palpably present in all the more advanced VortexHealing tools, increasing their power to generate transformation.

However, we can focus on this love by intending for VortexHealing to bring in just that quality. Then the divine love that is the inner fabric of VortexHealing also becomes the totality of its expression. The depth of love that comes through with this is truly profound.

Divine love helps you to remember what you are.

6. Bridging

When healing energy is being channeled, the channeler is acting as a 'bridge' between the healing energy and the receiver. What determines the quality of the healing will depend as much on the quality of the 'bridge' as the quality of what is being channeled.

Imagine that you are a churchgoer and that at the end of mass there are two priests who give short healings to the parishioners. Both priests, of course, will be channeling Christ for the healings. Both priests have been doing this for a number of years. One priest would rather philosophize about Christian concepts than do healings. He does the healings because he is required to, but his heart isn't in it. The other priest has fervently devoted his life to healing through Christ. When a parishioner comes before him, he deeply surrenders and opens his being, praying to be allowed to be a vehicle for healing through Christ.

In this example, there is little question as to who would perform the deeper healing. The devotion and surrender of the second priest would create a deeper bridge for Christ to come through, and the quality of the bridge makes a big difference. It determines how deeply the channeled energy will be brought into the receiver's consciousness and energy system.

A big part of what makes VortexHealing so powerful is the depth of the bridging that is built into the healing art. Although different individuals will have different levels of natural ability when it comes to bridging, the VortexHealing system naturally generates a deep ability to bridge—which deepens with each subsequent VortexHealing class taken—even for those students who have little natural ability in this area.

In addition to making in-person healings more powerful, this quality of deep bridging is what enables VortexHealing to be used so effectively at a distance.

7. Transmission

Most energy healing systems are 'taught'. There is a technique involved that the mind needs to learn and understand so the practitioner can duplicate it. (My first book, *Your Hands Can Heal,* is an example of this: it taught a simple energy healing system that could be 'learned' from reading the book.) VortexHealing is taught in a very different way—by direct consciousness transmission from the divine Source of the lineage. The 'teacher' of the class is simply the interface for the transmission. Of course, the teacher will convey whatever understanding is needed to work with the healing tools of that class in the most effective way. However, the teacher is not actually providing these tools. They are transmitted and integrated directly into the student's consciousness and energy system by the divine Source of the VortexHealing lineage.

This transmission process has three aspects to it. First, there is a direct transmission of the energetic healing tools. Second, there is a movement that evolves and accelerates the healer's energy system and consciousness. This enables the student to receive the healing tools as well as be a better vehicle for the divine energy and consciousness that will come through them. And third, there is the creation of a unique *bridge* in the student's system so that all the divine power that can be accessed by the student's system is also bridged very deeply into the receiver of the healing. With each level of class all three aspects of the transmissions go deeper, and there is a deeper and deeper bridging of Divinity through the healer's system. Because of this, even the healing tools that are taught in the Basic/Foundational class become deeper tools as a student progresses.

8. Healing by Intention

The magic of VortexHealing, in addition to its power, is that one can simply intend for the healing tools to clear a certain area or emotional issue, and Merlin's divine energy and consciousness go to wherever that is held in the person's system and creates transformation there. The healer, simply by intention, gets to play with this divine magic and to direct how it interacts. There is the sense of divine intention supporting your own intention, as long as it is appropriate.

As one student wrote:

> *For me one of the most profound results of working with VortexHealing has been that one can simply 'intend' something, in one's own consciousness, and, because of the support of divine intention, a response occurs 'out there', in external reality. This is quite astonishing, and, for me, it is an answer regarding the fundamental and true nature of reality: the primacy of divine intention over matter. This has changed everything for me.*

This process of intending/directing the flow of divine magic also sets up within the VortexHealer an active relationship with Divinity that only grows deeper over time. Even when healing others, the VortexHealer is thus deepening within their own path, opening to Divinity.

9. Magical Structures

All energy healing modalities channel some kind of energy and/or consciousness into the receiver, achieving whatever results they can from that. Starting with the second VortexHealing class, in addition to channeling and deeply bridging divine energy and consciousness, students can also channel what we call "magical structures". A magical structure is divine energy that has been made dense enough that it comes out in the form of golden-white threads that are full of divine intention. They can be used in various ways to strengthen organs and body systems, to re-structure the flow of energy and consciousness in a living or work space, to bridge certain qualities into a space, to improve the sound of a musical instrument, to emulate other kinds of healing modalities, and so on.

When structures are put into a body organ or system, they bridge a certain amount of Vortex energy into that system 24/7, helping to keep it strong. For instance, the first time I created a magical structure was for a friend who had psoriasis stemming from a sickish liver. I channeled the structure with the intention that it should strengthen his liver. The next day he told me that he must have gotten food poisoning the night before because his intestines were upset and he had diarrhea. I realized what had really happened: the divine structure had strengthened his liver enough that it was able to dump a lot of the toxins that had been stuck in it. This created the diarrhea as the toxins were flushed out.

When I channeled this structure, I had an intention for what it should do, but I had no idea what shape the divine threads should take or how it should interface my friend's energy system. Yet the divine intelligence of the lineage took those threads, manifested a unique divine energetic structure out of it, and interfaced it into my friend's energy system so that what I asked for could be accomplished.

These structures will last indefinitely, if appropriate. For instance, if a client has a weak system, these kinds of structures can be channeled into all of the client's organs and body systems, which will help to keep strengthening them indefinitely. While those structures are working in the background, the healing sessions can focus on whatever issue may be behind the weak system, as well as clear energetic blockages to improve the flow of energy through the pathways.

Magical structures can really illustrate just how magical VortexHealing is. For example, in public demonstrations, we will channel one into a room and intend for the room to take on a Feng Shui quality. Immediately the room feels like it is connected to nature, with a certain kind of flow going through it. Then we'll put a different intention into the structure, such as intending that it make the room feel like outer space. In a few moments, the whole quality of the room changes, and it feels as if you are sitting within a vast empty space. We can make the room feel like a desert, or like being at the sea, or like being by a waterfall, and so on, just by changing the intention we put into the magical structure. If we make the room feel like Mars, usually a few people in the audience start coughing.

In a similar manner, you can redecorate your house energetically with these magical structures. You could have your living room feel like the sea, your bedroom feel like Tahiti, and your bathroom feel like the moon. For those living in crowded areas, magical structures can create a filter for your home so all the chaotic mental and emotional energy from your town or city doesn't flow through it.

These kinds of magical structures are just the beginning. In more advanced classes, transmissions for all kinds of other divine structures are given—for the body, for homes, and even for large areas, such as towns and cities.

10. Emulation

VortexHealing's philosophy is that most healing modalities have something unique to contribute to our experience and understanding of ourselves and our universe. We appreciate these other modalities, and the magical power of VortexHealing enables us to emulate many of them. Our emulations, though, are controlled by divine intelligence, rather than a human mind. We don't have to be concerned about overriding the receiver's system or making a mistake in trying to balance it.

As one example: in the Basic/Foundational class, students can channel specifically into the acupuncture/meridian pathways—clearing, energizing, and harmonizing the pathways. Even with all the higher-level VortexHealing tools I have available, I still often use this acupuncture-emulation technique from the Basic/Foundational class when I am tired or feel out of balance. After 10-15 minutes, my energy level comes up and harmonizes. And when using this technique, I don't have to be concerned, as an acupuncturist does, about whether a particular meridian energy is too high or too low, whether it is stringy or empty, etc. I just channel Vortex energy to clear and harmonize all the pathways, and it gets done. Of course, this is an *emulation,* so it is not the same as acupuncture with needles. With needles, for instance, you can intentionally block energy flow as a way to block pain or for other purposes, which the emulation cannot do. So the needles can create effects that can't be re-produced by channeling Vortex energy. Yet the emulation also has benefits that the needles cannot create: it works through divine guidance, overall it is more energizing, and it can get deeper into the meridian system than can be accessed with needles. In addition, there is no concern about unbalancing the receiver's system with it, and you don't need four years of school to practice it.

Here is what an acupuncturist, who became a VortexHealing student, wrote about our acupuncture emulation:

> *VortexHealing affects the pulses in a very similar way to acupuncture, but qualitatively it can be much better than acupuncture. It's more harmonious, as the Vortex treats the body at a deeper level. The changes I get with VortexHealing are similar to what I would get with 5-element acupuncture if I were treating the body at spirit level. It has a deep, smooth, and harmonious effect on pulses—more than you would get treating with acupuncture on a symptom level or a general energetic level treating syndromes. Yet on a symptom level, it changes the pulses as effectively as 8- principle acupuncture.*

For example, for liver stagnation, the pulse will lose its wiry quality. Physical symptoms respond quicker than with acupuncture. There have also been times where the Vortex has gotten to things that acupuncture couldn't—as if the acupuncture took the system to some energetic wall but couldn't get through it, but the Vortex could go through that wall. I've been recently sensing the possibilities of channeling the Vortex directly into acupuncture points. At the very least, I've observed it works as well as needles, but without the pain. And I sense there are other possibilities, other benefits.

Other emulations are also possible. With the magical structures described above, students are able to access the Jin Shin pathway system, with the structures creating a bridge for channeling simultaneously into all the pathways of that system. There is a healing modality that works with the energy pathways that run through the core of the bones, keeping the skeletal system aligned. With VortexHealing's magical structures, students can focus healing energy so it creates a similar kind of flow through the core of the bones, realigning that level of the body. In a similar way, fascia tissue can be realigned, which is excellent for injuries. And those same students, working with a different healing tool from the second class (called "Merlin's Global Healing Grid"), can emulate "planetary pujas" and "dosha balancings", healing practices from India. They can also channel energetic crystals, which in later classes can be filled with frequencies, essences, and mantras. These energetic crystals can be channeled into organs and systems to help their functioning or can be used to create "crystal-gem balancings" that will work in the background as you sleep. When I do this at night, I wake up feeling as if my aura has been 'polished'.

In general, VortexHealing emulations will often substitute quite well for what they are emulating, but sometimes the original technique will provide something that the emulation cannot. For instance, using our craniosacral emulation, which releases tension in the cranial fascia tissue, I can often create more release of tension in my head than I would with a regular craniosacral session, but the original craniosacral technique can free up locked cranial sutures and twisted cranial bones, which the emulation can't do.

Perhaps our most magical emulation is that of psychological therapy. Often, when dealing with issues, it is not quite enough to clear identities and old conditioning, because the human personality still has its habits. Sometimes a conscious understanding or realization is needed by the personality for the whole thing to shift. Traditionally, psychological therapy facilitated this. VortexHealing recognizes this value, so we emulate it with a special transmission called Vortex Therapy. When this is channeled, Merlin finds a way to interact, at the subconscious level, with the consciousness of the personality. Magically, this does create a certain psychological movement at the personality level. Sometimes the person may still need a more conscious, conceptual understanding of their emotional process, which only face-to-face therapy can provide, but Vortex Therapy is often quite sufficient for this purpose.

II. Releasing "Karma Knots"

"Karma knots" are the focal points of the incarnational issues and identities, carried by the incarnational self from life to life. When a being incarnates into a new body, these karma knots show up as tiny dark spots in the center of the spine. I named these dark spots "karma knots" because they represent the karma for that individual in relation to that issue, and they contain lots of past-life memories, wrapped up like a knot into that little spot.

In the center of the karma knot is pure separation consciousness. Around it is a sort of bubble of webbing that holds both the consciousness of whatever issue that karma knot represents and all the most important, emotionally-charged, past life memories that support the issue. *The separation consciousness in the center of the knot is the true root of whatever issue that knot expresses*, for without it, there is no issue. For instance, the issue of being a victim requires a core sense of being a particular someone who is separate from everyone else. From a place of true oneness, there is no victim. As another example, anger may arise in a particular situation, but without that sense of separateness, there is no someone being angry, and so there is no issue, just the situational anger of the present moment. An issue requires a sense of someone-ness as a separate being. The issue *belongs* to that being.

Part of what makes VortexHealing so unique and powerful is that we are able to clear karma knots, even with the healing tools of the Basic/Foundational class.

The average number of karma knots for a human being is about 245. For perspective, it would be rare for someone to be truly interested in something as deeply spiritual as VortexHealing if they had more than about 60.

Here is one of my favorite karma knot stories:

> *I once did a treatment on an autistic, nine year-old boy. I could see that he was actually pretty far along on his spiritual path, for he only had three karma knots. I could also see that one of those karma knots was the root of his autism. I have always perceived autism as a karmic/emotional issue that generates a deep emotional shutdown. In this case, it looked like one of his last remaining karmic issues, which played out very strongly in his last life, had to do with avoiding his basic human emotionality. In the session, this karma knot released, and I told the parents that they might start to see some changes in the boy over time. Well, the changes started the next day. He had been afraid to walk into a room that was next to a room that dogs were in. The next day he went up to a dog and petted him. He had been afraid of heights, but now he started climbing fences. He became socialized enough to get into the school band. People who knew him were noticing these changes and were asking the parents if the boy was becoming normal.*

What happened with this boy illustrates just how powerful and important a karma knot is to an issue. However, to release a karma knot, you have to release that core spot of separateness, and only that which isn't separate can transform the consciousness of separateness. That's one reason that working with divine consciousness is so important when working on issues; divine consciousness operates from a place of oneness. In the Basic/Foundational class, when we channel Vortex for an issue, Merlin's divine consciousness knows if there is a karma knot related to the issue, knows if that karma knot is ready to be released, and knows how to transform that spot of separateness, awakening it to its true nature of oneness. When the karma knot releases, in that dark spot of separation consciousness divine light suddenly appears and the core of that issue is gone. The conditioning that supported that issue will still most likely need to be addressed, but with the living core of it gone, the leftover conditioning will be much easier to deal with.

12. Healing the Complete Issue

Our emotional issues are what cause us the most suffering. If we break a leg, aside from the initial pain, our suffering will arise out of how we react emotionally to the broken leg. If we have a background depression issue, then we may feel depressed by what happened and by the new limitations on our mobility. If we have a background anger issue, we may spend a lot of time being angry about what happened. Or we may feel victimized by it. Life will always pull our issues to the surface so we can encounter them, giving us the opportunity to transform them.

We all have an inner cabinet full of emotional issues; some of the issues are simply more obvious than others. The more hidden ones may only appear in particular situations that act to trigger them.

Earlier, I wrote that our emotional issues are truly 'comprehensive', which we can see by how deeply they catch us, and I went into some detail on this. The fuller picture is much more complicated because our consciousness and our energy systems are much more complex than what can be summarized here. Even identity is held in multiple places for an issue, on multi-dimensional levels. All of these conditioned places interact with each other and with the identity, with each part supporting the whole. *An issue is really a complex, interacting network of consciousness and energetics, on multi-dimensional levels.* So, if a key piece of conditioning or identity or enough smaller areas of conditioning are not cleared, what is left untouched will start to re-condition the other areas in the network, maintaining the sense of the issue in consciousness.

To fully clear an issue, you need to be able to address it and clear it sufficiently in all these different places, including the identity. You need to clear everything within the issue's network as well as the structure of the network itself. Eventually, to make the healing complete, you will need to go even further. You will also need to awaken the overall consciousness of separation that seeks to create identities, to reinforce the sense of itself in existence. Healing the complete issue requires healing more than the issue; it also requires healing your sense of separate self. You will need Divinity for that. You will need some way to bridge Divinity directly into the core of your being. That is what VortexHealing was designed to do: both heal the issue and transform that sense of separate self at its root.

13. Healing the World

When we talk about energy healing, we are usually referring to healing individuals. But all those individuals live in a world, and the nature of what is going on in that world, both locally and internationally, affects them. When most of humanity views life through the lens of survival need, it becomes much more difficult for you to be free of that perceptual constraint. If you are living in a town that is full of hatred, you will react to that, and it will tend to amplify whatever seeds of hatred exist within yourself. The VortexHealing lineage has always taken the larger view, and it has always used its divine healing powers to help the planet as a whole. To that end, it developed a specific healing tool, given to students in Magical Structures class, called "Merlin's Global Healing Grid", for working on *situations*. This can be used for personal situations, those affecting a workplace or local community, or even global situations.

Another kind of situation that Merlin's Global Healing Grid addresses is the buildup of energetic memory in a space or environment. Although clearing spaces of this kind of buildup may not seem all that important at first glance, it is an important form of healing. Whatever happens in a room leaves an energetic impression there. If negative emotional energy is given off in a room, it will linger there indefinitely unless it is cleared.

When someone walks into that room, they will unconsciously sense it. I'm sure that at some point you've walked into a room that had enough of a build up of negative energy that you couldn't help but sense it. If you don't sleep well in hotel rooms, it may be because of the energetic imprints of all the other people that have stayed in those rooms and in those beds. If you don't sleep well at home, it may be because of the energetic build up of stressful energy in your bedroom, from stressful dreams. Energetic imprints in spaces can also impact relationships. For instance, if you and your partner have an argument in the kitchen, the energy of that will stay there and you will both react to it, making it easier to have another argument whenever you are in the kitchen. It's best to periodically clear this kind of energetic imprinting from one's living space.

If enough negative energy builds up in a house, it can become what is called a "sick house", and children will have all kinds of problems growing up in it. Many VortexHealers have been called upon to clear up these kinds of spaces. Although we usually use Vortex energies to clear the enclosed spaces of homes or apartment buildings, Merlin's Global Healing Grid is needed to work on larger areas, such as towns or cities, which include outdoor areas.

Here is an example, shared by a VortexHealing student, which illustrates both how the energetic buildup in our environment can affect us personally, and how Merlin's Global Healing Grid can be used to heal the situation:

> A few weeks after I moved to my new home, I started to notice all these virulent, racist thoughts popping up in my head. They were completely foreign to my normal inner commentary, and for a while I couldn't figure out what was going on. Then I realized that I had moved into an area that has a long history of racial tension, and that some part of me must have 'plugged into' the memory of that tension still sitting in the environment. Once I identified the problem, I realized that Merlin's Global Healing Grid would be the best tool in my VortexHealing tool kit to address it, so I spent about 10-15 minutes using the Grid to clear the history of

racial tension in the local area. Immediately I noticed that the racist thoughts in my head were subsiding, and once I was done they all disappeared and never returned.

VortexHealers often connect as a group, using Merlin's Global Healing Grid to do these kinds of environmental healings on a larger scale. They also use Merlin's Global Healing Grid to transform issues within humanity as a whole, or within a particular country.

14. Energetic Development

The nature of VortexHealing is that its healing tools are given by transmission, which also means they are bridged by the divine Source of the lineage directly into the student's energy system. The level of development in someone's energy system is thus a limiting factor for how deep of a healing tool can be given. The transmissions, therefore, do not simply give those healing tools but develop the student's energy system so they can receive those tools. In addition to the healing that students receive from using VortexHealing on themselves, their energy systems undergo a continuing evolution and deepening with each class.

15. The Relationship Between Healing and Awakening

Healing modalities generally focus on healing, and spiritual practices focus on awakening. *VortexHealing uses healing to facilitate awakening, and it uses awakening to facilitate healing.* For us, healing and awakening are intimately related.

As incarnational beings, we are identified with all of the issues and emotional positions we carry from life to life. When we incarnate, we extend that sense of identity to our body, to our human mind, to our family, to our emotions, to different parts of our personality, and even to material objects, such as our cars or our homes. These all become part of our experience of separate self. In addition, our sense of lack drives us to become attached to things: to money, to status, to love, to a job, to particular possessions, etc. So we live at the center of a web of identity and attachment, drowning in our issues, and although we suffer from this, we continuously invest a lot of energy and inner beingness to maintain it.

When we start to use VortexHealing, we awaken the separateness and identities at the root of these issues. What we've invested in the issues is then freed, and it comes back to us as free energy and consciousness, helping us to remember our true being. As more of our web is transformed, more and more free energy and consciousness accumulate within us. This is the kind of transformative process that VortexHealing creates when it works on issues. It is not just doing healing; it is generating the ripening process that moves us towards spiritual awakening.

This also works in the other direction. Once spiritual awakening happens, healing issues becomes much easier, because the foundation for all of them has now been cracked open. In addition, every level of awakening creates a significant jump in the student's energy system, which then enables deeper healing tools to be given. These are then used to generate even more free energy and consciousness, creating more inner freedom, and the student can channel these higher-level tools to help others as well.

4   How VortexHealing® Heals

In this chapter, I'll describe the healing tools of the Basic/Foundational class in more depth. To understand how these healing tools work, though, I first need to describe the VortexHealing view of the nature of creation, as pertaining to what we call the "two webs".

The Two Webs of Creation

Since VortexHealing is a healing art, it needs a concise view of the nature of reality to know what it is healing. For instance, a doctor views a patient mostly in terms of biochemical and biomechanical processes. An acupuncturist views the body in a very different way, which involves energy flow through meridian pathways and how different 'elements' are acting and interacting in the body's system. A psychologist will focus on the emotional aspect of the person.

VortexHealing has its own point of view. We start with Divinity, which is ultimately all that is. All is Divinity, and so all is One. Creation exists because Divinity has become creation. Creation isn't a thing; it is Divinity expressed as patterns of consciousness, energy, and intelligence, arising within what we call the "two webs of creation".

The Vital Web: From a scientific viewpoint, the world is seen as a collection of atoms that interact according to certain physical and biochemical laws. Looking deeper, Einstein talked about a unified field of creation—where everything in creation is an expression of that field. Many ancient traditions would agree with that, and some have described that field as a web of lines of light. For VortexHealing, this is the "life web", also called the "vital web".

Everything we can see, touch, measure, and so on, is this vital web. In the VortexHealing map, it exists at 10 dimensional levels (with physical time and space being the first four of these dimensions). The basic energy of the vital web is vital energy, also called "life force energy", and its essential quality is vitality or livingness or *'am-ness'*, which the self identifies with and then experiences as *I am*. This web is not *within* creation; it *is* creation. And it is completely permeated with energy, with an elementary form of consciousness, and with a field of intelligence. From this point of view, everything in creation is a pattern of this web of vital life force, and the web lines that make up its complex structure become more compacted with each lower dimension until creation is dense enough to be experienced as physical.

Our body, as a particular pattern of this web, is designed so that when it looks out at the rest of creation (the rest of the vital web), what is seen is what we know as our familiar reality. Yet we know that animals and insects have different perceptual realities. We also know that even the physical part of our experience is just a perceptual construct: modern microscopes have shown us that the world is not really solid, that it is almost entirely empty space, and what we actually experience is constructed out of sensory input by our brains.

As a localized pattern of this vital web, our bodies are completely connected to it from all around our energy field. Yet all the web lines of our body come together at the navel, making that our body's vital energy center and our most focused connection to the web. Although we think of our perception as just occurring through our physical sense-organs, we also pick up information through this navel connection to the greater web.

As we interact with life—with the rest of the vital web—both our consciousness and the vital webbing of our bodies accumulate a unique history of experiences and become conditioned by it. Trauma, grief, anger, etc., are both patterns of consciousness and patterns of conditioning in the vital webbing of our bodies. As we'll see a little later in this chapter, understanding the vital-web structure of our body and how the navel functions with that will be very important, both for specific kinds of healing and for bridging VortexHealing more deeply when channeling.

The Divine Web: Although the vital web is creation, there is also a deeper web: the divine web. The basic energy of the divine web is divine energy. The divine web manifests the vital web, and thus it is the Divinity's vehicle for manifesting creation. Since vital energy is produced from divine energy, we can think of it as divine energy that has been 'slowed down' and densified so it vibrates as life force, and so it can be experienced by beings in creation as a sense of aliveness.

The divine web, therefore, is the deeper, underlying structure of creation. The 'outer edge' of the divine web is like the scaffolding upon which the vital web of creation is manifested. The divine web also continuously feeds the vital web energy and divine intention, maintaining creation and directing its evolution. In our bodies, there are major divine lines in our spine, coming out of the center of each chakra, and out of each hand and foot. The divine web cannot be conditioned by what happens in life, although as we'll see later in this chapter, divine lines can be broken.

Healing & the Webs: Knowledge of these webs is important for healing for several reasons: VortexHealing has a way to access the divine web to bring more energy into the vital web, energizing the body; a lot of healing for the physical body is directed at the body's vital web; and because it is possible, from trauma and from deep issues, for one or more web lines in our body to become broken. A broken line will create various symptoms, and those will be strong symptoms when it is a divine line. (See *Healing Broken Divine Lines,* later in this chapter.)

Basic/Foundational Class Healing Tools

The core healing tools that are received in the Basic/Foundational class are accessed through a divine energy/consciousness structure that is manifested by transmission within the heart of each VortexHealing student. This divine structure is called the "Vortex Wheel", traditionally called the Wheel of Life. It can only be created through a teacher of the lineage, whether that was given in this or a past life. That is how I was able to recover VortexHealing—I already had a Vortex Wheel from having studied this in two past lives.

The Vortex Wheel is actually a Divinity-based interdimensional Vortex, and it is the vehicle for accessing Merlin's divine energy and consciousness for the healing taught in the Basic/Foundational class. It is created out of Merlin's divine energy and consciousness. This is Divinity, which is our own deepest nature, expressing itself as a healing transmission within our energy system. As it does so, it creates a focal point that concentrates the energy channeled and makes it easy for us to access it. This takes the form of a divine vortex arising out of the spot where our heart chakra meets our spine, and opening out through the heart chakra into creation. It is called the Vortex *Wheel* because the only part of the Vortex that is visible, manifested in space and time, is what sits between the spine and the heart. Since the Vortex is much wider at the heart than at the spine, where it almost comes to a point, if you are looking straight at it, it looks like a wheel. In addition, when it is being used to channel Vortex energy, it spins, concentrating the energy. So, we call this transmission the Vortex *Wheel*. It is also described as an *interdimensional* Vortex because it bridges into all dimensions, enabling us to channel into them.

There are four things that a student can do with the Vortex Wheel: (a) channel the 49 unique forms of Vortex energy, (b) "Run Divine Lines", which is working with the divine web to energize various systems in the body, (c) channel "Merlin's Healing Essence", a healing transmission that brings in Merlin's divine consciousness and is also used to fix broken divine lines, and (d) channel a composite transmission called "Vortex", which simultaneously channels the previous three things we can do with the Vortex Wheel.

Below is a description of these healing tools that are packaged within the Vortex Wheel, as well as descriptions of a few other healing tools given in the Basic/Foundational class. For perspective, it's useful to note that my own early healings using VortexHealing (which I described above), could be done by any Basic/Foundational class student today.

A) The Vortex Wheel & Channeling Vortex: When a student accesses the Vortex Wheel and intends to channel "Vortex", these are all channeled simultaneously: all 49 Vortex energies, Running Divine Lines, and Merlin's Healing Essence.

B) The Vortex Wheel & the 49 Vortex Energies: Each form of Vortex energy has unique properties. Some of them bridge in particular emotional or spiritual qualities, such as love or peace. Most, though, are designed to do specific things in the energy system. (These were described above, in the section called *Energetic Specificity*, in Chapter 3.) The Vortex energies do this by interfacing the vital webbing that makes up the energy system of the body. When the energy is channeled into an organ, for instance, some of it goes to the vital webbing, clearing and energizing it, some of it works on the cellular level, and some of it clears and energizes the organ's energy pathways. Wherever Vortex energy is channeled in the body, it will energize, clear blockage, and clear conditioning in the energy system and in consciousness.

Vortex energy can be channeled into the system as a whole, into specific areas, or intended to go wherever most needed. It can also be channeled to clear and energize just the acupuncture/meridian pathways. Although one can simply channel all the Vortex energies together and let Merlin decide which one or ones to use, it is also fun to learn their different qualities. Here is an example where I used just one for a particular situation:

> *I was teaching a Basic/Foundational class. As all the teachers do in all these classes, I offered students "drug therapy". Some kinds of recreational drugs (as well as anesthesia) impact the brain and nervous system in a way that permanently impairs it. For instance, if I look at someone who has done crack— even once—it leaves what looks to me like burn marks in the brain that separate areas of the brain from each other. In this class, a young woman came up during a tea break who had once done crack. I channeled Violet Fire Vortex into her brain, because that is specific for inflammation, and I channeled until the burn marks seemed to disappear. The young woman's mother was taking the class with her, and later she came up to me and thanked me for "giving her daughter back". That one dose of crack had shifted something in her daughter's brain and personality; Violet Fire Vortex had healed that and brought her back.*

Vortex energies can be channeled one at a time, as in the above example. They can also be channeled all at once or channeled as part of the composite Vortex transmission, where they are channeled simultaneously with Merlin's Healing Essence and Running Divine Lines. They can even be used to clear spaces, such as homes, offices, schools, or hospitals. (See the section, *Clearing Spaces*, later in this chapter.)

C) The Vortex Wheel & "Running Divine Lines": As described earlier, not only does the divine web create the vital web but also continuously feeds it energy at every level—and that means to every strand of vital webbing in creation. Running Divine Lines is a healing tool that gets Merlin to feed or 'run' more divine energy from the divine web into the vital web. This creates extra energizing in addition to the Vortex energies, and it can be channeled quite specifically into a particular organ or system or wherever it is most needed, letting Merlin's divine intelligence decide. Running Divine Lines energizes in a very different, yet complementary way. If you imagine a strong emotional "charge" held in someone's liver, then in addition to the emotional component, the vital web in that area will become very congested and blocked, not allowing energy to flow through very well. If we channel Vortex energy into it to clear that charge, then it will start at the outer areas of the charge, working its way into the core. However, the divine web is already feeding the vital web of that area, both in the outer areas of the congestion and in the core simultaneously. By having Merlin add extra energy to what is already flowing into the core, it softens the emotional charge from the inside while the Vortex energy is clearing it from the outside. This makes its transformation much faster.

Running Divine Lines happens automatically when any of the main VortexHealing tools are channeled, but this can also be channeled on its own.

Healing Broken Divine Lines: Divine webbing is the 'infrastructure' for the vital web. As I wrote earlier, the most important divine lines in our bodies are in our spine, coming out of the center of each chakra, and coming out of each hand and each foot. Although the divine web and its lines cannot be conditioned, a divine line in the body can be broken in certain circumstances. About 1 in 50 people have a broken divine line— and they stay broken if they are not healed. If a line coming out of a foot is broken, it will have a dramatic negative effect on grounding. The chakras actually spin on the divine lines coming out from their centers, and if one of those chakra lines becomes broken, the chakra stops spinning, which effectively is like turning it off. That area will become energetically dead and the organs that depend on receiving energy from that chakra will suffer and develop symptoms. If a divine line coming out of a hand is broken, it will impact the sense of being able to connect to the world. If the main divine line in the spine is broken, it can cause death. (Vital lines can also be broken, usually from a physical injury. This can create a feeling of deadness in the injured area, but these lines usually heal on their own over time.)

The question may arise as to how a divine line, since it is divine, can become broken. The answer is that this is by divine intention, by Divinity cooperating with you in relation to a particular issue. Let's say you are about to be in a car crash. At the moment just before impact, something in you intensely craves escape. Because death feels imminent, that craving, whether consciously or unconsciously, is directed, by pure reflex, towards God. Something in you calls out, with or without words, "God!" or "Oh God!" to get you out of there, even if you're an atheist. Divinity may respond to the intensity of that, cooperating with your desire by breaking the divine line in one of your feet (usually the left one), helping you to get out of your body. After the accident, even if you are disturbed by the resulting ungroundedness, your desire to re-ground will not be as deep or intense as your original desire to get out. In addition, since it is no longer a matter of life or death, you most likely will not be reaching out to Divinity for re-grounding. So the line stays broken.

This is what happened the first time I taught a student how to fix a broken divine line:

> This student had been in a car accident, and even though she wasn't injured, she felt very 'out of body' after the accident, and this was very disturbing to her. She went from healer to healer trying to get back in, without success. Finally, she called me. I realized what had happened, but up until that point I had always fixed these lines 'manually'. At the time,

we hadn't developed a technique for VortexHealing to fix these broken divine lines, and she lived a few thousand miles away. I meditated on this, and after a bit, I realized how I could instruct her to use VortexHealing on herself to fix her broken divine line. After following my instructions, we spoke again. She said, "Almost instantly I felt a shift. I was back in my body again." After that she was fine.

Divinity can also 'cooperate with you' to break a divine line coming out of a chakra. Chakras both take in energy to feed local organs and are a vehicle for expressing emotional consciousness. Different emotional issues will show up in different chakras, and when an issue is deep enough, the corresponding chakra may have its divine line broken.

For instance, you may have a deep issue of emotional self-protection. This issue will be focused in the area of your solar plexus, which is the location of your third chakra, also called the solar plexus chakra. That chakra, along with its related organs, will hold a strong focus of the emotional charge of that issue. As the suffering from the issue goes deeper, you start to avoid feeling it. If your desire to avoid it and escape the suffering becomes intense enough, Divinity may cooperate with you by breaking the divine line coming out of your third chakra. Then you stop feeling what is held in that chakra and its related organs, as requested. But escape always comes with consequences.

Here is an example of the effects of a broken third chakra line and its healing:

I was giving a group VortexHealing in New York, and I noticed that someone in the room had one of these broken divine lines. I mentioned this to the group, intended for the line to be fixed, and then continued with the healing. A month or two later, I received a letter (people actually wrote letters instead of emails back then!) from a man who had attended that healing. He said that he had had stomach problems for many, many years, and had even learned a healing modality to keep the symptoms calm. The symptoms were always there, though; he had never been able to heal them. He was writing to let me know that from the time he went home after the healing, the symptoms disappeared and stayed gone.

When a divine line is broken, it can create major disturbances in the body. Most healers will spend a lot of time treating those disturbances, but they cannot get very good results without fixing the cause. Unless the line is re-connected, no amount of other healing or addressing other areas of the energy system will alleviate the symptoms. With VortexHealing, fixing a broken divine line is the easiest thing we can do. It only takes seconds, and then the symptoms tied to that typically clear immediately.

With an accident or short-lived traumatic event, the issue that breaks the line is usually gone once the event is over. However, if a line is broken because of a chronic issue, then if there is still enough desire to escape that issue, the line can be re-broken. Since this is more often the case with the breaking of chakra lines, when we encounter these it alerts us that other work may need to be done as well. But not always. Often, by the time the person discovers VortexHealing, enough work has been done on the original issue that the line maintains without any further work. This is what happened in the group healing I gave in New York: after a few seconds, the man's divine line in his third chakra was reconnected, and his symptoms immediately cleared up and stayed gone.

D) The Vortex Wheel & "Merlin's Healing Essence": Merlin's Healing Essence is the third transmission accessed through the Vortex Wheel. It brings in Merlin's divine intelligence and consciousness. Its focus is not on the energetics of the system but on the conditioned consciousness that is creating issues. So, in the earlier example of the emotional charge in the liver, while Vortex energies and Running Divine Lines are doing what they do at the energetic level to clear the charge, Merlin's Healing Essence goes straight into the core of the emotional component of the charge. It bridges divine consciousness into the conditioned consciousness and transforms it. When the conditioned consciousness is transformed, it is then easier for the emotional charge in the vital webbing to let go, while any clearing in the vital webbing makes it easier for the conditioned consciousness to be transformed.

Merlin's Healing Essence is the most critical transmission for working with emotional issues at Basic/Foundational level. It is also the key for clearing karma knots (described earlier), and it is what we use for healing broken divine and vital lines.

As with the other Vortex Wheel transmissions, Merlin's Healing Essence can be channeled by itself or as part of the composite Vortex transmission.

E) Merlin's Fire: This is a special transmission for burning out infections that students can only use on themselves. For work on others, they would use the different healing transmissions within the Vortex Wheel, including White Fire Vortex, an energy specific for infection. This by itself is very effective, yet when students have an infection, the simultaneous channeling of White Fire Vortex and Merlin's Fire will speed up the clearing.

F) Navel Hookup: In the section, *The Two Webs of Creation,* I wrote that all the vital webbing of the body in some way comes together at the navel. This makes the navel the energetic center of the body. Intuitively, this makes sense, because in the womb the baby is connected to the mother—and thus to life in general—by its navel. If that connection were to be blocked, the baby would die. After birth, the new human life is still connected to life through its navel, but it is an energetic connection now, not a physical one. Although we are connected to the general vital web from all around our energy field, our most focused connection is through the navel.

As part of the VortexHealing transmissions, Merlin created a way to use this natural, universal "navel hookup" to deepen healings. Since the channeler is already energetically connected through the vital web to whomever is receiving the healing, VortexHealing gives its students a unique healing transmission that enables them to temporarily amplify that connection for the time of the healing. It's like temporarily turning a one-lane road into a superhighway so more vehicles can travel through;

we turn the innate navel connection into an energetic superhighway so more divine healing energy can pass through, from channeler to receiver. The actual effect is not just that more healing energy passes through but also that it bridges the energy deeper into the receiver's system. As in the story of the two priests told earlier, it is not just what is being channeled, but also how well it is being bridged.

We call this our "navel hookup" transmission; but it doesn't create the energetic connection between healer and receiver; it just focuses it. Whenever the VortexHealer stops channeling, this amplified hookup instantly stops as well.

In each class after the Basic/Foundational class, the ability to bridge into the receiver and into the vital webbing of creation is deepened. So, when an advanced Vortex student channels the same Vortex energy received at Basic level, it has a more profound effect, effectively making it more powerful.

G) Meditations: Meditations can be an important part of the healing process, and different meditations are valuable for different purposes. In the Basic/Foundational class, we teach several different meditations. This enables the student, through meditation, to facilitate any of these movements: (a) to relax out of the movement in their consciousness, so they can rest deeper in their natural inner being, (b) to help bridge their awareness into their issues, which helps the issues to release, (c) to de-stress, which naturally helps improve health, (d) to open their "spiritual heart", and (e) to bring in divine presence, which creates more opening on a deep level, helps to awaken issues, and helps to deepen the relationship with Divinity.

All in all, these VortexHealing meditations bring that magical, transformational power that is part of our lineage more deeply into the core of the student's being and life.

H) Grounding Cords: Babies are born with a "grounding cord" that is a part of their energy system. It helps them to 'ground' and feel connected to the earth. It also strengthens and supports their overall energy system. At conception, the livingness of the earth bridges to the womb to create an energetic connection with the new earth-body that is growing there. That energetic connection grows as the fetus grows, and when the spine and energy system are sufficiently developed, it becomes a grounding cord. The cord starts in the center of the earth, comes up into the spine, filling the whole spine, and interfaces the navel and heart. The interface to the heart helps create a heart-connection with the earth and with nature.

The problem is that in industrialized countries, most people have lost their grounding cord by the time they are a few years old. This occurs because we have learned to objectify the earth rather than feeling our organic connection to it. We ignore the feeling-sense of that connection, and over time the energetic aspect of it, in the form of our grounding cord, breaks down. Children then grow up surrounded by adults without grounding cords, and they quickly pattern that and drop their own. In doing so, they lose the energetic support the cord provided, as well as the emotional support that comes with an organic connection to the earth. Since our grounding cords connect us to something larger than our individual egoic selves, without them we become even more isolated and separate, and that supports all our issues and all the suffering that arises from them.

In the Basic/Foundational training, students have their grounding cords re-established. Once that is accomplished, they can also help others to re-establish their grounding cords.

l) **Clearing:** One of the magical things that can be done with Vortex energies is clearing negative energies from enclosed spaces: homes, offices, schools, hospitals, shopping malls, etc. Even whole apartment buildings can be cleared—and in less than a minute. As long as the space being cleared is within an enclosed structure, the whole space can be cleared, no matter the size. An aftereffect of this kind of clearing is that the air feels lighter, fresher, and easier to breathe. It even feels energized. In addition, there can be other unique aftereffects, depending on the particular Vortex energy being used. For instance, if one chooses to clear the space with Merlin's Love Vortex, then afterwards a subtle quality of divine love will be left in the space, like a perfume filling a room. If it is a bedroom that is being cleared, one might choose Dream Blue Vortex or

Merlin's Peace Vortex. One could also choose a combination of different Vortex energies, to combine different subtle qualities for the space. The VortexHealer can choose which Vortex energy or energies to use, or have Merlin choose.

For open spaces, Merlin's Global Healing Grid (given in Magical Structures class) is used, as described above, in the section, *Healing the World*.

Advanced VortexHealing® Classes

Although the Basic/Foundational class gives the student a complete set of healing and transformational tools, VortexHealing is not this single class. It is a complete system of healing and transformation that accesses deeper and deeper parts of the energy system and consciousness as classes progress. In each of the more advanced VortexHealing classes, the healing tools from the Basic/Foundational class deepen and new healing tools are given that get to new areas of the energy system and deeper dimensional levels of consciousness. In *Chapter 6: The Human Package*, you will read some examples of what these more advanced healing tools can address.

The other aspect of healing addressed in the more advanced classes is the need for awakening out of our sense of separate self. Although we want to heal our issues and our bodies so we can be free of our suffering, the deeper desire is for wholeness, to more fully experience what we truly are. However, this deeper desire often manifests as the desire to heal issues, for we believe that if only we could heal our issues then we would be whole. Of course, healing our issues is an important part of our healing process, but the separate self can never be whole. It is a different kind of healing that brings us to wholeness; it is the healing that releases this sense of separate self. That's why VortexHealing, as a divine healing art, sees awakening as a fundamental part of any being's ultimate healing process, and why it is a central part of what it offers to its students.

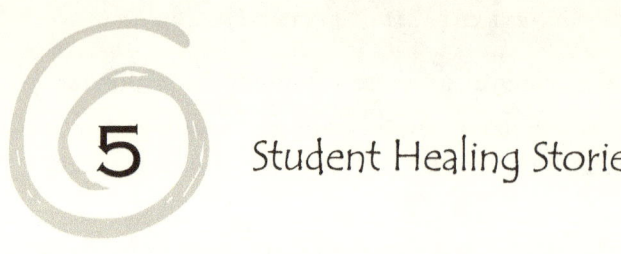

5 Student Healing Stories

The following stories, all reported by VortexHealing students, were picked to illustrate the wide range of healing that can be effected with VortexHealing. Many, many more such stories can be read on our website (*www.vortexhealing.org*). Just click on "Stories" in the top menu bar.

A man who's about to have a neck tumor extirpated starts to receive sessions to relax before the surgery. He has many fears, insomnia, tachycardia, the feeling of choking, difficulty swallowing. In the first sessions, the symptoms diminish. He indicates he feels better. He takes six more sessions and has a consultation with his doctor to go over the studies and to coordinate the day and time of the operation. The doctor checks him out but can't find the tumor. The studies are re-done and it appears that there's a remission of the tumor. He continues to have sessions once a month.

I had a big success treating viral-based chronic fatigue. A young lady of 18 had been a sufferer since 11 years old and after three sessions it has completely cleared from her system. I did the sessions over six months ago and the symptoms have not returned.

Also a lady who has had headaches every day since she was a teenager (she is now in her fifties) was symptom free after a few sessions using energetic intervention [an advanced VortexHealing technique] and channeling to work on issues and blocked energy lines to her head.

For 27 years I had eye pressure (glaucoma). After I discovered VortexHealing, I began to treat my eyes every day. The pressure started to normalize. I stopped using the drops that I had been prescribed. The pressure normalized completely, and all the checkups done in the seven years since then indicate normal eye pressure.

I want to tell you that Omega energy [from an advanced VortexHealing class] also worked wonderfully on tulips. I got a bunch of them from a client. Two of the flowers started straight away to hang down. After using the energy they stood up right again and still are for the sixth day. Nice!

I've been working with a client for a few weeks now. She had a large fungal mass behind her heart that was pressing on her lung and causing her to cough incessantly, making it impossible even to sleep. Once it was diagnosed, I started working on her, hitting the physical as well as the emotional sides of it. A couple of weeks later, a follow-up x-ray showed that the growth had diminished in size, and today a new CAT scan showed no growth whatsoever. They want to do another follow-up in three months, but for now she has a clean bill of health - all without surgery or toxic anti-fungals.

I'm sending you another magic story. Actually these things happen every day, but sometimes they are so evident that it's fun to tell them.

My friend asked me for WD-40 for fixing the electric rear window of his 11 year-old Korean SUV. It was fully open and there was no way to close it. He tried all day millions of times and it would not close. We would have to disassemble the panel of the door and lubricate somewhere to see if that fixed it. Quite a hard job and we had no tools and no light. It was a dark garage.

So I took 15 seconds to make a structure [from Magical Structures class] with the intention of lubricating whatever was stuck. Kind of nurturing a dry bearing or gear. 30 seconds later the window began working. We could close it. Amazing!!!

I treated a woman by distance last week. She phoned me the next day to say she felt better. She sent me a check and wrote this, 'It is incredible the difference to my back. I could not walk—the pain was unbearable, now it is almost gone. I could not walk or even get out of bed. I was crawling to the bathroom for days. I am now fully mobile. It is a miracle."

As an equine veterinarian, I have used VortexHealing for over 20 years on horses, both in the US and in Panama. The horses are very grateful for the healing, and stand very still to receive the healing. The results vary from good to phenomenal. A few horses had their lives saved. I have also used the healing on some other animals, such as dogs, with success as well.

VortexHealing healed my moderate depression (without any relapse) and gave me back my sense of humor. Amazing!

The 67 year-old client I was treating for the 'incurable' bone marrow disorder went for another clinical test last week and his blood was pronounced 'fine' by the nurse who is still puzzled by it all! He is due for another check up in three months' time, which should be his last check up. He is going to continue on a maintenance-type plan monthly with Vortex.

Needless to say he is 'over the moon' with his recovery—he thought he was going to die and was told that he would be on blood transfusions for the rest of his time. I have used different Jewel-level techniques [advanced level VortexHealing class] with him, including working with the cellular consciousness of his bone marrow cells and also, to begin with, I used Energetic Intervention [an advanced VortexHealing technique].

I tried the VortexHealing re-orienting technique on a child who was having problems at school with reading and writing. When I channeled it to him, the energy was really pumping. A few weeks later I spoke to his mum and not only was he reading but he was enjoying it too. Before the healing, this boy could barely stay focused, let alone read. His mum also mentioned that he seemed a lot more settled and centered in himself.

I was healing my uncle's cow, which was dying of some kind of disease, and not responding to any veterinarian medications. The cow received two treatments, 20 minutes each, of divine VortexHealing from me. The next morning the cow was healthy.

When I first started VortexHealing training, I was a wreck: physically, mentally, emotionally and spiritually. I was working in an ego-filled world as an executive in broadcast television and suffering from the stress of chronic fatigue from an undiagnosed gluten allergy. During the second class, I sat up and said to myself, "I am an energy healer," with absolutely no concept of what that meant or how that was going to transpire. As I found out, the process of awakening was and IS chaotic, challenging, frightening, confusing, painful, dark, light, beautiful, liberating, mystical, Divine, peaceful, joyful, blissful and life changing. Fast forward to the present day where I am using what I have learned and am still learning to help clients transform and evolve into their own true potential. Looking back, all I can do is marvel with infinite gratitude at the Divinity that brought us all together... It can only be called one thing – "magical".

⊚

I am constantly surprised at the power of VortexHealing - on myself, on others and with the surroundings. Opening to the Divine through VortexHealing is both a privilege and a miracle.

⊚

During a medical examination, my son was diagnosed with eyelid carcinoma, a diagnosis later confirmed by another professional through tools (not biopsy). He was sent for surgery to another specialist, but it would be 20 days before this specialist could see him. In the meantime, he received Vortex constantly, several times a day. At first the injury worsened rapidly, but then it began to improve. When he had the new medical consultation, his eyelid was normal.

⊚

On April 12th, I found out that my 79 year-old mom in Sweden had a tumor in her bladder (seen on an MRI). I did a distance VortexHealing session for her that day. She was going to do surgery (laparoscopy) on April 24th. When my mom was on the surgery table, the tumor was gone!! No surgery needed.

⊚

We were called at 5 am to come immediately if we wanted to say our last goodbyes to my grandmother, as the doctor said there was nothing that could be done. Well, Merlin disagreed and I found myself doing all this karmic clearing while standing at the end of her bed. She came back to her senses and got way more vital and communicative.

Once we got back home from seeing my grandmother, I shared with my parents what I did during the visit. About a week later, my dad received a phone call from my grandmother's sister. In the midst of her bewilderment, she was making a casual comment "I don't know what happened....how is this possible", to which my dad said: "Well, I don't know what is possible and what is not, but this is what happened," and went on explaining what I had shared with him. There was absolute silence at the other end.... And my grandmother ended up living another 2.5 months.

I have a client who has been coming to see me for over 11 years now. She first presented with a fertility issue. She and her husband had been trying to conceive for the past six years. I gave her three VortexHealing treatments, and then I met her husband and he had a VortexHealing treatment as well. She was pregnant after one cycle and they now have four children ranging from 11 to 2 yrs old. They all come together now for regular updates.

My little girl cat Maggie will remind me if I forget to clear and put VortexHealing structures into her food. I have three cats, and make them each a small plate of canned food and take it into my healing room to feed them there rather than underfoot in the kitchen. If I forget to clear the food and put structures in, she leaves the food and follows me back to the kitchen and gives me a "look". She then leads me back to her plate and waits until I "fix" it. She is so funny. Have to love those little affirmations of what we do.

A man was taken to the ER at the hospital where he had had a transplant of his abdominal aorta. His body was rejecting the transplant and I was called in the middle of the night by a sobbing niece (she herself is a prominent doctor, who even writes articles for a medical magazine in the US), saying that she feared her uncle would die before dawn, due to his critical state. I worked on him long distance, trying to make the transplanted organ look like the rest of his body. The mimic worked out well. He's back home and feeling alright. His body stopped rejecting the organ.

A friend had insomnia for months and tried everything under the sun but nothing seemed to work. I finally convinced him to have a treatment. I did half an hour and I could not believe it when he told me a week later that he had been sleeping!

A lady who had ovarian cancer came to see me just before she went into hospital for the operation to remove it. I gave her a full healing treatment and broke the timelines connected to her womb and other womanly bits, and she felt much calmer. She had a slight tummy ache and a bit of a bleed, but felt much better about the thought of losing her ovary. When she arrived at the hospital and had an examination, the tumor had gone and she was sent home!

A woman of 26 was suffering from fear of death, to the extent that it had almost turned into panic attacks. Her mother asked me to give her a couple of sessions while she was here on holiday. She has gone back and feels great.

I had a teenaged patient who was so electro-magnetically sensitive that she couldn't be near microwaves, fluorescent lights etc., and each time the sun did a burp (solar eruption), she broke out in hives, was blind with migraines, had intense body pains etc. She hadn't been able to attend school for years and had hardly any friends. She was extremely smart and talented, and her dream was to study graphic design/animation, but often could not bear to be in front of a computer.

After five sessions, she is feeling normal and symptom-free—for the first time in her life— and is going off to college on her own and catching up on living the life of a teenage girl!

I feel very grateful for the opportunity to experience the VortexHealing path—both as a practitioner and as somebody who is seriously interested in releasing layers and layers of accumulated inner pain, and becoming lighter and more aware and awake. I was drawn to learn this art after taking ten sessions with a VortexHealing practitioner, during which a fibroid that had been sitting on top of my uterus for years simply disappeared. This miracle has changed my consciousness and my life. If something like this can happen, anything miraculous can happen.

What I now simply love to do most is to give VortexHealing sessions. The energies that are then flowing through me are incredibly sweet, for the lack of a better word, and put me in a blissful state, much more so than I have ever experienced in any other way, including meditating in Indian ashrams in the presence of enlightened masters.

Seeing the miraculous shifts and transformations in people who receive sessions is often even more rewarding. And if I didn't already know about the magical effects such a healing session can have, I would have become a fan after each session I received from other VortexHealers. In fact this is what gives me the courage to live a rather adventurous life.

Each time I went through what felt like severe heartbreak—after divorce, the breakup of a love relationship, or the nearly unbearable physical pain caused by issues that are flaring up in these collectively very intense times of revolution and regime change where I live, in Egypt— VortexHealing has so totally shifted me out of it, that I can hardly relate to how I felt before the session. It keeps amazing me.

6   The Human Package

We think of ourselves as a single, unified being. This sense that we are unified comes from two sources: we experience the same sense of self internally, and we project that same sense of unified self onto others. Even when we (or others) behave erratically or have unexpected reactions to events, it doesn't shake our sense that there is a single unified being at the center of that.

Yet this seeming unity masks the fact that we are also a multi-dimensional, eclectic collage of disparate parts. The masking of that certainly helps our sanity, but for healing purposes, it is better to understand the organization and functioning of all the separate parts and how they interact, to give us our unique experience of this journey.

The Journey & the Incarnation: We are not just human beings; we are *incarnational* beings. We have lived thousands and thousands of lives, starting from long before we became human. As we journeyed, not only did we accumulate more personal history, we evolved a complex incarnational personality that over time accumulated issues, karma knots, identities, and experiences of trauma. All of this drove us deeper into the experience of struggle and separateness until we could go no further. Then, from a deeper place within us, a quiet voice whispered, "There must be more to life than this," and we began the journey back to freedom, back to Divinity itself, our original true nature. If you are reading this book, you are well on the return part of your journey, but you are still carrying all that old personal history, along with whatever trauma, karma knots, issues, and identities remain. You are still living within the structure of the incarnational personality that was created around all that history. You brought it all with you into your new human body, and by various mechanisms it imprinted itself into every organ and body system, every energetic pathway, even into your DNA, and into all the different aspects of your new human consciousness.

At the same time, all the history, issues, and identities of your biological ancestors, going back millions of years, have been passed down from generation to generation through their DNA. DNA is essentially a biological survival mechanism, and so all that ancestral memory about the process of surviving is hardwired into our DNA. Your body was created out of that and is now saturated with it. As a result, this survival memory and all that came with it conditions not only every cell of your body and all of its vital webbing, but also all the aspects of your psyche, including your incarnational consciousness.

This merging of conditioning, between the incarnational being and the new body, happens on multi-dimensional levels, and has been deepening since conception. So, by the time you are born and everyone is adoring the cute, bubbling baby, everything is already in place. Your psyche and body are already deeply locked into all the history, issues, and identity inherited from both your personal and ancestral history. It just isn't very obvious, for two reasons: the new cells of the body have not had time to get heavily imprinted by all this yet, and the body is full of a certain kind of "essence of livingness"—what Chinese medicine calls "pre-natal Jing"—which radiates qualities of innocence, purity, and a sense of light and aliveness. Together, these two factors hide what is going on deeper within the body and psyche.

For most individuals, their core inner drama of struggle (to avoid suffering and death) will emerge, in one form or another, as the main focus of their life. That could show up as a struggle for food and shelter, a struggle within one's job or relationship, or simply a struggle to be healthy or happy. Often, it is a mixture of these (although much of the suffering within all this is suppressed from conscious awareness). Whatever form it takes, because all experiences will be perceived through the frame of the underlying struggle, life will tend to continuously reinforce the conditioning of the drama being experienced at that time, solidifying it and the experience of being a separate, struggling self. But if you are on a path to inner freedom in this life, then your journey back to wholeness will create another focus that will compete with the original one. Now, instead of simply playing out your drama, you will be looking for a way to become free of it. You will search for a way to become free of your karma knots, free of the issues and identities that lock you into separation and suffering, and free even of your sense of separate self.

It would be much easier if these issues and identities, or even your sense of separate self, were just 'in your head'. But they are also imprinted and conditioned into every one of your cells and energy pathways, into all the unconscious areas of your psyche, and even into your physical brain. If an issue or identity is not cleared *systematically* from all the areas where it is held—as well as its roots—then the issue will still 'resonate' in your body and psyche, and it will still trap you.

The ability to do this kind of *systematic healing* is part of what makes VortexHealing so powerful. This kind of healing can also make VortexHealing seem complex. Yet it is not VortexHealing that is complex; what is complex is the human consciousness and energy system that is being healed. If someone is hired to clean a multi-story house, they only bring a vacuum, some kind of soap, and a roll of paper towels; but if a list were made of all the areas they needed to clean in that house, it would seem very complex. Most healing modalities simply open the windows, letting in some fresh air. What this doesn't do is clean the dust out of the carpets, bookcases, drapes, or under the furniture; it doesn't clean the grime off the tile or toilets or sinks; it doesn't clean the windows or wash the kitchen floor. If there is a mold issue in the kitchen, opening the windows will freshen the air and feel nice for a little while, but it won't deal with the issue.

A form of systematic healing that has the power and depth to get into all the nooks and crannies of the body and psyche is critical to freeing oneself from an issue. We have to also keep in mind the large picture: the person receiving the healing is on a journey. The journey is not simply about their presenting issue; it is also about getting free of their overall situation of struggle and suffering. This ultimately means bringing them back to unity and wholeness, to their true inner being.

The rest of this chapter is designed to flesh out the overview given in this section so you have a larger sense of what we are addressing when we do healing on a human being. This means giving you both a sense of some of the different areas that VortexHealing can heal and transform, as well as presenting the larger context for these specific healings in terms of our journey.

Structure of the Human Package

A) Two Personalities: We have a sense of ourselves as particular human beings with various identities, emotional patterns, likes and dislikes, etc. However, our basic human personality is really made up of two distinct personalities, each a gestalt of many mini-personalities that express in the same space of our human consciousness. One is your incarnational personality; the other is your genetic one.

1. **Incarnational Personality:** The being you experience yourself to be is rooted in your incarnational history. You have been this being throughout your entire incarnational journey. This is the basis of your sense of personal self. Yet your incarnational personality is a gestalt of many pieces, many mini-personalities, each with its own self-identity, emotional positions and issues. When you incarnate, you bring all that with you, carried both in your incarnational consciousness and your incarnational 'body'. You then extend your incarnational sense of self and identity to your new physical body and all the ancestral material it contains, turning all that into new experiences of self. To support this process, your incarnational self also grows what we call "karmic webbing" out of its karma knots, which grow this into various energetic levels of the new body. The incarnational being then uses that webbing as a vehicle for expressing its consciousness and issues through the new form. All of your issues will have karmic webbing that will need to be broken down.

Note that there are also deeper dimensional levels of consciousness and conditioning at play in the background of the incarnational personality's psyche. Unfortunately, it would add too much complexity to this book to explore those deeper levels here. More details can be found in my last book, *Awakening Through the Veils*. For the purposes of this book, it is enough to know that advanced VortexHealing classes provide the tools to work on these levels, as they do ultimately need to be addressed to unfold a spiritual awakening that is true inner freedom.

2. **Ancestral/Genetic Personality:** Your genetic history, carried in your DNA, has its own personality, derived from the personalities of your

ancestors. That personality, like your incarnational one, is a gestalt of many pieces of personality, each with its own self-identity and issues. (Interestingly, because the incarnational being is present at conception, the consciousness of its own personality becomes part of the new genetic one, mixing with the ancestral material.)

When you incarnate, you identify with your body, your body's personality, your body's sense of separate self, and all of the body's ancestral history and issues carried in the genetics. Since this is all then experienced as self and arises in the same field of human consciousness as your incarnational personality, the fact that it remains a distinct personality is usually not conscious. Instinctively, we identify more consciously with our incarnational self and suppress much of what we experience from our genetics. We do this because our genetic personality typically holds much more suffering. All that memory of death and dying, of desperate struggling to survive, of starvation and illness, etc., is a lot to handle. Although our incarnational personality experienced these things in different lives, it innately knows that it survives death and disease, and so that kind of memory doesn't weigh so heavily on it. In addition, it is connected to deeper dimensional levels of self. These levels of self are still trapped in separation, but they hold much less suffering and have access to deeper dimensional levels of light, which makes us feel freer there.

So we push much of the pain in our genetic personality out of our awareness, and we use the positive feelings the body can generate— feelings of pleasure and aliveness—as an additional camouflage. However, this suppression turns our genetic self—along with suppressed areas of our incarnational self—into our 'shadow'. Camouflaged or not, much of the clearing we need to do for our core issues needs to be done on this shadow self; much of our deepest suffering is held there. We cannot move deeply into inner freedom without dealing with our shadow.

It's easy enough to become aware of your shadow personality. First, look at what a friend is presenting to the world as their personality, as their self. Then tune into their body, but look past the general sense of aliveness there; just sense the kind of emotional self that is held there. The two personalities will be very different. The one they are consciously identified with is held in the spotlight; the other one still has their identity in it, but it is held in the shadows. When you can sense these two personalities in someone else, try to sense them within yourself.

B) A Complex Body: The body is made of vital webbing, so when there is a physical injury with no emotional component, then the healing work is solely focused there, in the vital web of the physical body and the consciousness that permeates it. But that vital webbing isn't just a chaotic mass of energy lines. It has been densified and organized into many different levels of bio-physicality: atoms, molecules, cells, tissues, organs, and various kinds of body systems. The general consciousness within vital webbing then becomes organized as atomic consciousness, molecular consciousness (including genetic consciousness), cellular consciousness, organ consciousness, and so on. There is also brain consciousness, consciousness within the energy pathways and chakra consciousness. All of these areas and levels of consciousness interact and are part of a larger bodymind consciousness. When there is a physical injury with no emotional component, it is not so important to pay attention to these levels; we just channel into the body and the divine energy and consciousness is taken to whatever level of vital webbing needs it. Emotional issues, though, including diseases with emotional components, are a different situation, because they generate emotional conditioning in the consciousness of each of these areas of body structure, as well as in the other areas of consciousness to be covered in this chapter, and in the two personalities described above.

For instance, if someone has anxiety issues, most energy-channeling healing modalities would use a general shotgun approach, channeling to simply "clear the anxiety". However, the anxiety will be cleared much more deeply by clearing all emotional conditioning from each level of bio-physicality and consciousness that it is held in, which is what we do with VortexHealing. (We don't bother with the atomic level.) This kind of specific clearing focuses the transformational energy much more intensely at each level, enabling a fuller, deeper clearing.

C) Personal & Universal Self: Our basic identity is that we are an individual being, separate from everyone and everything else. This is our 'self'.

Although we also identify with our body, our personality, and our emotions, our deeper identity is this sense of being a *personal* self. All of our other identities arise from this egoic sense of personal self.

Our sense of personal self arises from our sense of separateness. This is the sense of 'I' and 'me' as separate from you. In spiritual writings this is often referred to as "ego". Our sense of self is extended into everything we identify with—whether that is our body, some aspect of our consciousness or personality, or something external, such as our family or our car. Spiritual awakening is the process of losing our sense of 'I' and 'me', since this sense of separateness is what keeps us from experiencing our deeper oneness. There are many levels to the sense of self (described in my book, *Awakening Through the Veils*), and each level will correspond to a level of spiritual awakening.

Universal self is the underlying foundation for the sense of personal self. It is the general sense of self that pervades all of life, all matter, and all consciousness—vital webbing consciousness, genetic consciousness, and incarnational consciousness. A plant doesn't have an individual self that can reincarnate, but through its connection to universal self and the vital energy of creation, it expresses a sense of *I am*. That general sense of *I am* pervades everything, even rocks. Our body has this consciousness of universal self, but it also carries an individual sense of self, derived from both its genetic personality and from the conditioning it takes on from the incarnational self.

Because this universal sense of self is the foundation for the personal sense of self, people think of it as their "higher self". But even universal self is something that is generated in consciousness and contains the sense of separateness. *What we truly are is beyond consciousness.* If we must use the word "self" to refer to what we truly are, calling that "True Self", then keep in mind that True Self has no sense of self in it—it is the no-self self, or 0-Self. It is a bit ironic, but true nevertheless. (For referring to what we truly are, I prefer terms such as 0-Self, Divinity, and Awareness/Being/Light/Love.)

Often, when people go into a mystical state of being "one with everything", they have simply dropped the sense of personal self and moved into a state of universal self. (Walt Whitman's long poem, *Song of Myself*, is an example of this; it is not true awakening.)

Understanding the role of self is important, because self generates identity and issues, and it acts like glue, holding those issues and patterns in place. Once we know that our sense of self is at the root of all of our issues and all of our suffering, we have a choice: we can go on living as we have always lived, or we can seek to become free of the prison of self; we can become spiritual seekers.

Although we want to heal our issues and bodies so we can be free of our suffering, the deeper desire is for wholeness, to more fully experience what we truly are. However, this deeper desire often manifests as the desire to heal issues. We believe that if only we could heal our issues then we would be whole. But although healing issues is part of the larger healing process, the separate self can never be whole. It is a different kind of healing that brings us to wholeness; it is the healing that releases this sense of separate self. That is why VortexHealing, as a divine healing art, sees awakening as a fundamental part of any being's ultimate healing process, and why it is a central part of what it offers to its students.

What we are is beyond the sense of self; we are the free awareness that has lost itself within this experience of being a particular someone.

D) A Localized Intelligence Field: The VortexHealing point of view is that there is a massive field of intelligence that pervades creation, which is derived from divine intelligence. Our human package has a localized expression of that field, which holds the blueprint for how everything in our human system is constructed and functions: our energy system, genetics, cells, personality, consciousness, emotional issues, attitudes, thought-patterns, and even beliefs, on many dimensional levels.

This field is thus the foundation of our life. From a healing perspective, some of the deepest roots of our issues will be held here, as blueprinting and patterning that programs our emotional consciousness and bodies. This programming is not written in stone, however, or it could not change with evolution. The more advanced levels of VortexHealing can transform it.

In the bigger picture, the VortexHealing view is that this field is also a vehicle for humanity's evolution. Although our genetics are programmed primarily for survival and carry eons of that kind of memory, our view is that divine intention is slowly creating a transformation in our Intelligence

Fields that will eventually bring a new kind of program into our genetics and consciousness that is based on love.

Fundamental Conditionings that Pull Us Deeper into Suffering & How VortexHealing Addresses Them

From the beginning of our experience of separateness, we begin an incarnational journey that takes us deeper and deeper into separateness and suffering, accumulating issues along the way. At some point, we start working on these issues as part of a larger process that is mostly invisible to us until we get near the end: the movement towards spiritual awakening. Below, we'll explore some different ways that our issues are held in our system, keeping us in struggle and suffering, and we'll look at how VortexHealing transforms them as part of its larger intention of 'ripening' the person for true awakening.

A) Karma Knots: Our karma knots are the roots of our incarnational issues, carried from life to life. The deepest part of a karma knot's structure—its true foundation—is the spot of pure separation consciousness at its center. (See *Releasing "Karma Knots"*, in *Chapter 3*.) We begin our incarnational journey with just one karma knot. As we deepen in separation, more are created, reflecting the complexity of our developing emotional drama and the number of issues we can bring to it. Humans have, on average, about 245 karma knots.

Every one of our major issues will have at least one karma knot at its root. That issue will most likely be reinforced by the ancestral history and identity carried in our genetics, and by the parents we had, since we tend to be given parents who have issues similar to the ones we are working on. (It will also be reinforced by the blueprinting for it in our Intelligence Field.) Yet because our basic identity lies more with our incarnational history than our genetic one, the core of the issue will still be the karma knot or karma knots that relate to that issue. This is where our basic sense of separateness resides within the issue; this is the foundation of the issue.

An issue cannot be resolved without the clearing of its karma knot. In the example given earlier in the book, of the autistic boy who started to undergo radical behavioral changes when the karma knot at the root of his autism was released, we see how fundamental a karma knot is to our issues. Once a karma knot is released, it cannot grow back.

Karma Knots & Awakening: Before anyone can awaken, all their karma knots must be gone. With the losing of the last karma knot, a certain level of energetic and consciousness development has been achieved. This needs to develop further for one to become truly ripe for awakening, but losing all one's karma knots is a key milestone. In fact, there is typically an experience of more inner space and freedom, along with less reactivity, after the last karma knot is released.

Because the divine Source of our lineage is deeply focused on our spiritual evolution and awakening, by the time a student has finished their third VortexHealing class, all their karma knots have been released. For context, though, no one would be interested in taking a VortexHealing class until they reached a certain point in their spiritual journey. As I wrote earlier, anyone who would actually take our Basic/Foundational class would already be at a point where it would be rare for them to have more than about 60 karma knots. Yet most people only clear one or two karma knots, if any, in their entire life, and that usually happens at the moment of their death. So to clear up to 60 karma knots in three classes is pure Grace.

With the healing tools from the Basic/Foundational class, you can also help others to clear their karma knots.

B) Identity: Karma knots hold the root identities for the incarnational being. Yet the incarnational body will also mirror the incarnational consciousness and create its own identities. On the level of the physical body, the ancestral consciousness that is carried through the genetics will also hold identities (called "genetic emotional patterns"). From both the incarnational and ancestral consciousness, the root identities for issues then grow into other areas of the human psyche and energy system, creating local identities there. For instance, when an issue imprints its conditioning into an organ, the 'organ consciousness' can create an identity in relation to that issue. This happens in chakras and in the brain as well. Each of these identities maintains the sense of the issue in consciousness. With VortexHealing, we release all the identities associated with an issue.

In the bigger picture, having an identity with something means that you are experiencing that as yourself. You have moved from the beingness and freedom of your True Self to experiencing yourself as some localized emotion, image, or body sensation that you hold as self in your consciousness.

So from the VortexHealing point of view, releasing an identity not only frees you from a particular support for an issue, it brings you back to what you are. It creates inner freedom and wholeness. It is part of the larger process that is the goal of VortexHealing: awakening you to your true nature.

C) Trauma: Trauma is different from other emotional issues in that the energetic and emotional charge associated with it will be very dense, very intense, and have a lot of energy bottled up in it. Trauma tends to pull us instantaneously and very deeply into our experience of separateness, leaving us struggling and suffering. If the trauma is not cleared, then it persists in the consciousness and takes on a life of its own—it becomes its own piece of personality continuously communicating its pain to the rest of the consciousness. It can also be carried into future lives as incarnational memory.

Because of the density and focus of the energy involved with trauma, releasing this kind of conditioning needs a healing energy that can be concentrated and bridged very deeply. Although the regular VortexHealing tools can clear both emotional and physical trauma, the lineage has evolved special tools designed for just this kind of energetic and emotional condition. This enables the release to go much more quickly. Here are four of them, which illustrate four very different ways we approach the trauma:

Breaking TimeLines: This works on the idea that both our body and our emotional states are continuous in time, and that continuity acts as a kind of glue, maintaining our current state of being. So to change something in our state of being, a shortcut would be to 'take it out of time'. This transmission enables the VortexHealing practitioner to do just that. It enables them to temporarily put organs, chakras, meridians, body systems, or a particular trauma into a state where it oscillates between manifestation in time and non-manifestation. In this state, without the glue of time holding it fixed, the divine Source of the lineage can quickly empty that system of history and trauma, which can create instantaneous dramatic results. Here is a simple example:

> *A student had fallen off a low cliff some six months prior to my seeing her. The broken bone in her arm had mended, but from the trauma, the tissue of the arm was still swollen and her shoulder had locked up, so she could hardly move her arm. Although she was having physical therapy, it was not getting to the core of the trauma. After breaking the timeline of her injury-trauma—which only took a couple of minutes—she had almost full range of motion. The change was instantaneous. And by the end of the day, the swelling had completely disappeared.*

Depending on divine intention, breaking a timeline can help heal a physical or emotional trauma, or it can release conditioning in a particular system, improving energy flow and health there. It can also, more dramatically, shift the course of a person's life, moving it from one direction to another. The latter, more dramatic effect is rare though; I have only seen that occur twice during a healing session.

Replacing Vital Webbing: Whenever there is a very dense, concentrated emotional or physical trauma charge, the key will be at its core. That is the point of greatest focus of energy, without which the rest of the charge either falls apart or becomes easy to clear. The charge will be melded into some spot of vital webbing in the body's energy system.

Instead of trying to release the charge from those strands of vital webbing, this technique simply replaces those strands of vital webbing melded to the core of the charge with 'brand new' vital webbing. Imagine having a black ink stain that won't wash out from a white wool sweater. This technique, which we call "Replacing Vital Webbing", would be equivalent to replacing the stained strands of wool with brand new ones.

Replacing the core energetic charge of the trauma weakens its overall focus and power, and then whatever is left is easily released. Only the highest level of VortexHealer can do this, as the depth at which Merlin's divine energy and consciousness can be accessed at that level makes this possible.

"Waking Up" the Trauma: For emotional trauma, the core of the emotional charge will be rooted in the experience of separate self, in the egoic sense of 'I' and 'me'. This acts as a kind of energetic glue, holding the trauma in place. Yet just as the divine consciousness within the VortexHealing tools can awaken the separation consciousness within a karma knot, at the higher levels of VortexHealing it can also awaken this egoic glue within traumatized emotional consciousness. With the egoic glue gone, what is left of the emotional charge becomes very easy to release, for now it is 'empty'; there is no one—no egoic self—occupying it.

Clearing Fixations: If something sufficiently traumatic happens to us, our consciousness can fixate on it and stay stuck there. These fixations generate a certain kind of emotional structure in consciousness, and that structure holds the fixation in place. When a fixation is deep enough, it becomes embedded in the incarnational consciousness and is carried from life to life. The body can become fixated from trauma as well. Fixations can lead to fixated or addictive behavior patterns, and they distort both the consciousness and energy system. With advanced levels of VortexHealing, we check for fixations when we do healing on issues. If they are present, we break them down.

Clearing Fascia & Biochemical Pathways: Fascia is the connective tissue that permeates muscles, so the fascia pathways hold the muscle-memory of the trauma. Trauma also creates biochemical changes, as the energetic of the trauma imprints into the energy fields of the biochemical interactions. After clearing the core of the trauma, we clear it from the fascia and/or biochemistry to release the body tissue's memory of it. All the healing tools of the Basic/Foundational class, including the 33 Tissue Vortex energies, help clear trauma from the fascia. This creates biochemical changes, but to work directly on the biochemical pathways, a deeper VortexHealing transmission is needed. Clearing the fascia and biochemical pathways will help both recent and very old trauma. Here's a short example from a student:

> *I began channeling to clear fascia pathways for my entire right arm & shoulder mechanism, releasing trauma and injury from tissues: WOW after only 30 minutes, what a difference! Burning needle sensations are gone and that constant deep ache went from ten to a two and I could lie on my back again. Relief after nine months!*

D) The Brain & Nervous System: Interestingly, the brain and nervous system is often neglected in energetic healings (and conversely, are mistakenly seen as the *only* things that need to be shifted in other modalities). Yet the brain and nervous system will reflect whatever is going on elsewhere in the system and becomes conditioned by that. If we ignore the brain and nervous system, then the identities and conditioning there will maintain the issue in consciousness and will even start to re-condition the issue in areas of the system that were cleared.

There are five ways that the brain and nervous system hold conditioning: (a) in its cellular consciousness, (b) in its biochemical pathways, (c) in the networking pattern of the neurons, (d) through identity, and (e) in the microtubules within the neurons (which scientists say hold memory as 'quantum vibrations'). At higher levels of VortexHealing, we work on each of these, both in the brain and nervous system.

Although the brain and nervous system aren't the root of an issue—the issue existed before the being even inhabited that body and brain—changes there can have a significant immediate effect. Here is an example:

> *I was doing a session on an autistic child. I 'transformed the cellular consciousness' of his brain—and I could see things rearranging in his brain as I channeled to create this shift. His mother told me that the next morning, for the first time ever, he told her a joke. He had laughed at jokes before, but*

he had never told his own joke. Something had obviously changed in his brain.

E) Blueprints: Blueprints are used to build houses and office buildings. They are also used by Divinity to build human bodies and lives, and to support our involvement in specific issues. These blueprints all exist at higher dimensional levels.

Intelligence Field Blueprinting: Our local Intelligence Field is an expression of the massive field of intelligence that pervades all of creation, through all dimensional levels, and it holds the deepest level of blueprinting and programming for everything going on within us. Because it takes into account all of our issues from our incarnational existence, as well as from our ancestral history, *all* of our issues have a foundation here, on a very deep level. At the highest level of VortexHealing training, we can transform what is held here, and when we work on an issue, this is where we start.

Since there is an aspect of this field that comes from and pertains to our incarnational being, whatever is not transformed there will be continued in the next life. So when we work on an issue in this Intelligence Field, not only are we creating more freedom from struggle and suffering in this life, we are also working on our overall incarnational journey.

Specific Blueprints: There are also various kinds of more specific blueprints, created for very specific purposes. These exist at higher-dimensional levels (but not as deep as our Intelligence Field), and they are designed to guide the emotional life of a being. For instance, at conception, Divinity may create one of these specific blueprints for the key issue you need to work on in this life, which will make your experience stronger in relation to this issue, forcing it to become a major area of focus in your life. Bringing it into focus is just the first half of the journey for that issue; at some point, it becomes time to release it. Yet that can be difficult when there is a higher-dimensional blueprint holding it in place.

Another kind of specific blueprint that guides emotional life is a 'parental blueprint'. This kind of blueprint is not actually held by the parent but by the incoming newborn child. The blueprint creates a kind of groove in the child's consciousness—out of all the different ways that child might relate to its parent, the child tends to follow the groove, setting up a relationship with that parent that matches the blueprint. The parent will automatically react and respond to the way the child is relating to them, reinforcing the pattern and setting up a particular relationship. Out of all the possible relationships that could have been, the blueprint pretty much guarantees that a particular one will be played out. Since our relationships with our parents tend to get projected onto everyone else, these blueprints are also critical for all our relationships.

The way I discovered these upper-dimensional blueprints illustrates their power:

> *My mother was visiting. At this time in my life, my relationship with her was not very good, and I found that every time she walked into a room that I was in, something in me tightened up and sort of growled inside. After noticing this a few times, I sat down to meditate on it, to clear whatever it was. It would seem to clear, I would go back into the general living space, my mother would come in, and there was the same reaction again, as if the healing I had done on it counted for nothing. This repeated several times. Each time the reaction would seem to clear, it would instantly come roaring back when my mother came into the same room that I was sitting in. Finally, as I meditated with this yet again, I tuned into Merlin and asked what was really going on. I was shown a higher-dimensional blueprint that was holding the reaction in place. I used VortexHealing to clear it, and once again went into the general living space. When I encountered my mother there, the reaction was gone. Completely gone! I was quite shocked. And from the place where I was no longer being held in that old relationship with her, I experienced her in a new way, seeing her in a new light. I had an appreciation for her as a being that I never had before, and I felt a compassion for her that I had never felt before.*

Even if your parents are no longer alive, your present relationships are still being constrained by these old parental blueprints. At the higher levels of VortexHealing we release these, as well as issue-blueprints and genetic ones. At that level, it takes at most two minutes to release all the blueprints connected with an issue. This opens the space for the rest of the issue to be cleared, and the suffering that goes with it.

F) Black Holes and Spots of Non-Existence: If a fear of annihilation or unbearable emotional pain becomes focused and dense enough, it can form a compressed point of emotional contraction that is dark and dense enough to look like a "black hole". When these exist, they are usually found somewhere along the spine, although they can form in a chakra or organ. Only about one in three people have these. Once created, they are carried by the incarnational body and consciousness. Then in each new physical body, an area of vital webbing is created that is so compressed that very little is consciously seen or felt inside of it. Yet the pain/terror/ annihilation fear inside of it is there and will cause the personality to compensate for it, typically with a certain amount of withdrawal from life.

When a black hole goes even deeper, when someone starts to crave non-existence deeply enough to avoid their pain, even if unconsciously, the black hole morphs into what we call a "spot of non-existence". This is the deepest place of suffering that we create on our incarnational journey, and we will carry it with us until it is transformed.

Once this kind of spot arises, it will become, from the background of the person's consciousness, the center of their emotional life. All issues will revolve around it in one way or another, and will continue to do so, life after life. If one of these is found and the student is at the level to work on this, it is the first issue we work on. We can't release the conditioning within one of these spots because the vital webbing has actually been damaged by what is being held there—it has gone into an almost dead state. Instead, we use the technique called Replacing Vital Webbing (described above in the section on Trauma) to simply create new vital webbing that is undamaged in the core of that spot, which then enables the conditioning left in that spot to be cleared. These spots of non-existence are found in about one in seventeen people. However, one in eight people will have a *mini*-spot of non-existence, which is less powerful of a focal point for emotional consciousness.

We can treat a black hole in the same way we release a spot of non-existence, but it can be cleared with other high-level VortexHealing tools as well.

Here is a student's experience of releasing her own spot of non-existence:

> *Since birth, I've always felt fractured, distant and not really present to and with my life. Vortex has been quite a relief and help in so many powerful ways and aspects...but I've still felt this 'distance'. But now, !WOW! since releasing my 'spot of non-existence', I've felt like I've come alive again for the first time ever!!*

G) Our Ancestral Convolutions: At some point, to become free of those genetic/ancestral issues of struggle and suffering, you need to be able to address the consciousness of the DNA. This is very difficult for a healing modality to do. Even VortexHealing needed specific healing transmissions to enable us to do this. Yet we can now engage this level very deeply. In addition to how this kind of healing can impact the physical body (I wrote earlier about how I was able to improve my Gilbert's Syndrome, a genetic condition), it can have a major impact on our core struggle and survival issues. Here is an early experience of mine with this:

> *When I first used VortexHealing to clear one of these kinds of issues in my own genetic consciousness, it was a bit of a shock at first. Because part of my consciousness had always been locked in survival, when some of it suddenly disappeared, it felt a bit strange at first, as if a part of myself was missing. My mind, which had the habit of looking for that survival energy, kept thinking that I ought to be stressing, even though it was suddenly clear that I didn't need to do that now. After awhile, though, my mind caught up and something deep in my psyche relaxed.*

H) Our Energy Bodies: Just as we have a physical body, we also have a number of "energy bodies" that occupy the same space as our physical bodies but are made up of different densities of "subtle tissue". Each energy body is a vehicle both for having and expressing certain kinds of experience. We have (a) a spiritual body, which is a vehicle for certain kinds of spiritual experience, and which is impacted by deep loss and events that make us lose faith in Divinity; (b) a mental body, which holds mental patterns and attitudes, and creates a mental framework for our issues; (c) an emotional body, which holds the 'juice', the emotional 'charge', of our emotional issues; (d) an etheric body, which is an important part of our energy field's interface to the world, so boundary issues, self-protection issues, and co-dependency issues show up here; and (e) a karmic body, which enables the incarnational body to interface the physical body and express into it all of its incarnational issues and karma knots.

VortexHealing is able to work on all these bodies, including clearing karma knots, with the Basic/Foundational class.

I) Needs of the Personality: Sometimes, even after releasing the core of an issue and most of its supports in consciousness and the energy system, there is still something that needs to shift on the personality level for the issue to transform. That something may be a certain conscious understanding or realization or letting go that still needs to happen. Without that, the suffering around that issue will continue in spite of all the other release that has happened. So VortexHealing developed the emulation described earlier, called Vortex Therapy. It is an advanced VortexHealing technique that works surprisingly well to help the personality have that final 'something'.

Whenever we've done deep work with an issue, we always use Vortex Therapy to help complete the movement through the personality. We can use this for the genetic personality as well, after deep genetic emotional work has been done.

J) Situations: Although all of our suffering comes from our own issues, often our issues become tied to external situations. Resolving these situations won't in itself heal the issues it activated in us, but doing so is a form of healing and does alleviate suffering. For working on situations, we have a healing tool called "Merlin's Global Healing Grid", which is given in our second class, Magical Structures. Although this healing tool can also be used for personal issues, it was designed to work in a larger way—on work situations, relationships, family dynamics, and so on. It is used to work on global situations as well. This aligns with the historical responsibilities of this lineage. Its work for healing and transformation has always been multi-focused: for individuals, for humanity, and for the planet as a whole.

If you are going to have surgery, you would want your surgeon to understand the complexity of what is being operated on. In the same way, the more we can focus on the specifics of what needs healing, the deeper we can go. An analogy is to think of using a flashlight in a large, dark room. If you widen the beam, you see more of the room at one time, but you can't see what is hidden in the shadows. If you narrow the beam, which concentrates and brightens it, you can see those places more clearly. With VortexHealing, the analogy would be that we use both wide and narrow energetic beams. For something like "energizing the system", a wide beam works better. For clearing deep emotional charges and identities, a wide beam doesn't have the focus; a more laser-like beam, or an energetic tool specifically designed for that situation, is needed. What is also needed is a comprehensive picture of how a human energy system and psyche are constructed so the healing tools can be used most effectively.

VortexHealing has all of these, and it also has a 'journey-wide beam', a view that illuminates the individual healing in relation to the receiver's overall incarnational journey and works on both. This increases the inner freedom within the being, ripening them towards awakening. Without awakening, you can become more peaceful, but you never experience peace. You can become freer, but you never become free.

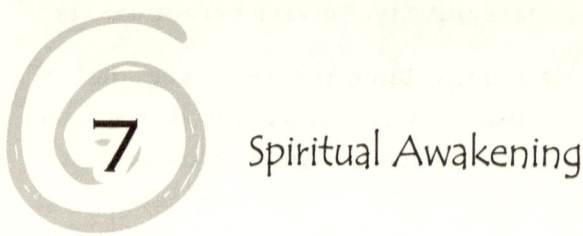

Spiritual Awakening

Basic Awakening

In the previous chapter, I wrote about the personal and universal self. Our sense of self is our most basic identity, the source of all our other identities. The personal self, though, has a deep existential issue: it is not the source of itself and so it can be annihilated at any time, making its very existence fundamentally unsafe. This is reinforced by our identity with our body, for which death is a certainty. As a result, our self cannot live from a place of true openness or peace, but rather continually compensates for its basic insecurity: it tries to control, it gets anxious, it gets angry, it gets aggressive, it gets defensive, it resents, it feels sorry for itself, it struggles, etc. Over time, these become fixed patterns of reactivity and identity, and we live our lives within the web of human drama and the issues they create. A spider creates a web to catch its dinner, but although we spin our own web, what gets caught in our web is ourself. We become lost in our personal drama of personal self. We may at times be happy in that drama, but we are never free of the drama itself or the basic identity of personal, separate self that keeps it all in place.

In addition, our sense of separate self keeps us isolated and robs us of a direct connection with life. We maintain our sense of self through constant self-referencing in our minds, continuously creating stories about our experiences with our self as the main character. So we end up living in these stories about our self instead of in life itself, and we miss the freedom and the oneness of our true beingness.

The only way out of this self-made mental prison is through spiritual awakening. Awakening is not about making our drama more manageable but about true freedom from the drama itself and from the boundaries that isolate us. Some people imagine this as transcending life or going to a higher plane of existence. But that would just be an avoidance of life. Life is here and now, and you are here and now, so if you are being true to what you are, there is nowhere to go. The whole range of manifest and unmanifest existence, from Divinity to egoic self, from formlessness to physicality, is all here now. Awakening isn't about hiding from life; it is about being present in life, but in a way that is not trapped by issues, by identity, or by the experience of separate self. Awakening is freedom. Awakening is returning to the truth and heart of what you really are.

We cannot go from our experience of separateness to full and complete awakening all at once. We are woven so deeply into our multi-layered web of drama and delusion that our energy systems couldn't handle the shock of this kind of movement. So there is a progression in awakening; we wake up one level at a time. The fantasy is that awakening happens and then it is all done, that we have reached the end of the road; but with our first awakening, we have only reached the end of the evolving-towards-awakening road. The journey continues, but now it is from a new, awake place. It is a new beginning.

The first level of awakening, which I call "basic awakening", releases the core sense of 'I' that sits in your heart. Although your mind is filled with thoughts of 'I', your basic sense of 'I', if you follow it inside, tracks to your heart. Since the heart holds the basic sense of identity, it makes sense that your basic sense of 'I' is going to sit there. And with basic awakening, that 'I' is going to disappear. Since the word "awakening" can mean different things to different people, VortexHealing defines exactly what it means by this first level of awakening: the sense of 'I' in your heart disappears.

As one student wrote after this awakening:

> When looking inside my heart I thought 'something is missing'. Something that had been there didn't seem to be anymore. I started to experience a new kind of well-being and peace in my heart that hadn't been there before.

People have all kinds of experiences that they like to think are awakenings, but most aren't. Most of those experiences are just expanded ego states, and most of the rest are simply a momentary taste of something deeper, and then the moment passes. Even when someone has the lovely experience of having merged with all of creation, that is an expanded ego state. A separate someone is needed for the experience of merging. There is nothing wrong with this kind of experience—it's one of the most satisfying experiences a self can have—it's just not awakening. Before my own awakening, I had a series of "samadhi" experiences, which are usually defined as states of transcendent bliss. At the time, I thought this must be what awakening is, but every time I went into this kind of bliss, it only lasted for a few moments. Then I came back to my familiar egoic reality. I asked a spiritual teacher, named Papaji (H.W.L. Poonja), why I couldn't stay in that transcendent bliss state. He said to me, "For every going, there is a return." In true awakening there is nowhere to go; you are simply here. If you have gone into some state, then at some point you are going to return. That isn't true awakening. Being awake is being here and now, but free of the identity of separate self. Rather than feeling expanded or transcended, the overriding quality of the basic awakening movement is most aligned with the words 'empty' and 'peaceful', in the sense that it feels empty of a familiar egoic sense of self, and this creates a sense of being at peace. When this is true awakening and not just a taste, then the experience will be permanent.

If basic awakening is losing this sense of 'I', then what is this 'I' and where does it come from? It comes from Divinity creating an experience for itself in which it forgets its wholeness and enters a state in which it knows itself as an individual, personal self. At first, this egoic self is like a tiny seed, only existing in higher dimensions, and then it is 'grown' into lower dimensions and densified, until the incarnational self is created. (A more detailed, step-by-step explanation can be found in my book, *Awakening Through the Veils*.) From there, the sense of self grows more identities, accumulating karma knots and eons of experiences and conditioning, digging itself deeper into the experience of separateness, getting lost in struggle and suffering.

However, no matter how deeply into separateness you go, this sense of separate self, of 'I', is ultimately just an experience that your own deepest nature is having. Ultimately, the awareness within the egoic self is divine awareness; it is just 'veiled' within the multi-dimensional maze of identities that it has created for itself. Awakening is the loss of the sense of separate self, but it is not the loss of what you are. Awakening is the shedding of false identity, the shedding of what veils you from your true nature, until all that is left is what you have always been.

Although some traditions teach that 'I' is just a thought or concept, it is clearly something more fundamental. For divine awareness to veil itself from itself, to become 'I', something more substantial than a thought is needed, or the false sense of 'I' would too easily break down. To hold the sense of 'I' in place, a construct is created in consciousness that creates a localized sense of self and veils us from our true nature. That veil sits in the center of our heart, which is why our core sense of 'I' is experienced there. I call this veil our "Core Veil". In basic awakening you awaken out of this illusory sense of 'I' created by your Core Veil, and your Core Veil breaks down.

To lose your Core Veil—to awaken out of it—a ripening process must first occur. One part of that process, for instance, is losing all of your karma knots. Once the Core Veil breaks down, the particular I-sense and identity it has created disappears with it.

This can bring in a deep sense of peace and natural beingness, free of the egoic sense of 'I', making it seem as if everything has changed. Yet the awakening doesn't eliminate the old mental and emotional conditioning (even if there is now no sense of 'I' inside of it). The Core Veil is not a package of conditioning but rather the original seed for it. Releasing the Core Veil does not eliminate what has grown from it, but rather changes your relationship to it all, for it is no longer yours. Whatever issues and conditioning you had going into awakening, whatever thinking patterns and attitudes you had, will be there on the other side of awakening. So the experience after awakening can also seem to be that everything is still the same. This is the paradox of basic awakening: *everything changes and yet everything remains the same.* You inhabit the same package of conditioning, but your relationship to all of it has changed. The emotional reactions you always had to particular situations still arise, but they no longer grab you in the same way because there is more inner space now, more freedom, and the fundamental sense of what you are, even in the midst of these reactions, has changed.

This typically creates confusion, at the very least. And with the old conditioning arising but no longer experienced as 'mine', the confusion can seem overwhelming at first.

Yet for different individuals, there can be a wide range of initial responses. There can be fear, or loss, or disorientation. There can be laughter at the absurdity of having believed that this 'I' was you. There can be a sense of relaxed beingness arising from the awakeness. Sometimes it is all of these, sequentially or even simultaneously. This is not what we expect from our spiritual fantasy of what awakening will be like, but awakening is never what we expect.

The confusion only lasts for a time, though. The deeper sense of peace eventually sorts it out, making it possible to give up the egoic survival struggle and all the suffering that came with it. It becomes possible to let go of your maze of false identities and rest in what you are, instead of always needing to *become* something, to define yourself. Awakening ends your old journey of someone trying to get somewhere, and a new one begins: a journey of opening to oneness, of inner being unfolding itself to itself. Yet this new journey still happens through the experience of humanness.

There are a great many spiritual fantasies about what will be experienced with awakening. The most common are: a permanent state of bliss, complete freedom from all suffering, great psychic powers, and complete transcendence. If you examine these expectations carefully, though, you see that they are more of a wish list for an ego trying to escape its suffering. They have nothing to do with true awakening, which is the falling away of the sense of personal 'I'.

However, there is also a tiny thread of truth in some of these fantasies in that these qualities do emerge to some extent in advanced states of awakening. If I am a spiritual seeker and I meet someone in such a state, I imagine that this is what I will experience when I awaken. In addition, even before my actual awakening, I may have had a moment where I experienced a taste of the perfection and grace that is true reality. These experiences feed the ego's desires, giving it hope, and great expectations are generated with respect to awakening. But three major problems stand in its way.

The first is that these advanced states of awakening are very different from the first level of awakening. I like to say that with basic awakening, you come out of the false identity you believed you were, but you have not yet begun to awaken to your true nature; that comes later, as a deeper awakening—if you keep going deeper.

The second major problem is that our perception of someone in an advanced state of awakening is filtered through the experience of a separate sense of self. That egoic self tries to imagine itself having an experience that matches the one it perceives—in someone where there is no egoic self. But an egoic self cannot imagine what it will be like when it ceases to exist. All it can do is imagine itself in the middle of some kind of blissful or transcendent experience, and such an imagining will always be utterly false. The egoic self can never be in the middle of an awakening experience because awakening, by definition, is a *no-I zone*. Bliss may arise at various points, but the ego will not be there in the middle of it.

It's as if you are dreaming that you are a gorilla. Within the dream, the gorilla becomes aware that it is dreaming and you wake up. At that point, the gorilla simply disappears. The gorilla may have had the idea of waking up, but it is part of the dream and disappears when waking actually happens. The gorilla didn't wake up; the dreamer did. The only difference with spiritual awakening is that when you awaken out of the sense of 'I', the world around you is still the same. With the dream of 'I' gone, everything changes, yet everything remains the same.

The third problem with the ego's fantasy about awakening is that awakening is a phenomenon that happens within our humanness. It begins to free us from our human drama, but we still have to live and express that through our humanness. You can't escape from your humanness or from dealing with your existence. What you may be able to experience in a moment of peak intensity is not something that you can live continuously. Your experience will always be a human one. Yet with awakening, you start to shift from a human being seeking freedom, to freedom itself being human.

My book, *Awakening Through the Veils,* goes into detail about the phases of awakening and provides help for seekers to get from wherever they are to releasing their Core Veil. (*Visit www.vortexhealing.org/books.*

htm for more info on this book.) There are also a number of articles I have written about awakening, which can be found online at *www. vortexhealing.org/articles.htm.*

Snapshots of Awakenings from Students

Here are a few short descriptions from students about their own basic awakening. There are more and longer stories in the next chapter, including stories about later awakenings. These short snapshots were selected because they illustrate different possibilities for what might be experienced when awakening first occurs. Yet there is a common thread that becomes apparent when you read these: a sense of a new beginning, or of some core boundary, limitation, or suffering that has broken down and given way to freedom.

The first story describes a student's overall process as it unfolded after her awakening. Of note in her description is her emotional process with it, and how the awakening ultimately impacted many different areas of her life, including some physical issues she had. Awakening can bring up all kinds of suppressed emotional material because there is now a new openness and space, which makes it easier for this kind of conditioning to emerge:

> My awakening process has brought me to places of extreme emotional release including terror and bliss. My family relationships and friendships and even meetings with strangers are much clearer and more loving. I am much more relaxed and all of my allergies and digestive problems have cleared. I still get confused about intimate relationships. I have a deep connection with nature and an even deeper connection with Merlin. When I am still, then the Truth sings from my heart.

The next story talks about the overall process, post-awakening, and how other people's perception of you may change:

Losing my Core Veil was the first day of the rest of my life, which becomes less mine and more real, more free and more simply love with each awakening class. On the way home from class I called my parents and my father did not recognize my voice on the telephone. It was so profound he even called my mother to come and listen to me, and they told me the tone had completely changed!

Another student shared a similar story: that her husband, for the first time ever, didn't recognize her voice when she called him after her awakening. The change in the voice is actually a common experience.

In the next story, the student shares his experience at the moment of awakening and points to what underlies the change in voice phenomenon:

For me, I almost didn't notice it when my Core Veil finally dropped away during the Core Veil class, but I do remember that the entire class gasped when I first spoke because my voice had changed so dramatically. It sounded different to me, too. It was as if a 'container' around my voice that had always echoed my words back to me had disappeared. I never noticed that container before, but once it was gone, I felt like my words just reverberated out forever into emptiness. Then I looked inward for the sense of 'I' in my heart that I had been meditating on for years, and when I asked myself once again, "Who am I?" instead of feeling my familiar 'I', I felt emptiness—and laughter! The very question was now absurd and hilarious to my heart. Instead of an 'I' there, I felt stillness and joy.

This student's story describes the awakening experience in terms of identity:

I felt something like a small ball drop out of my midsection, and I immediately started laughing. Such a tiny little weight, and yet so much of what I thought of as identity had been bound up in it. I entered an odd state for about three days in which I felt like I completely lost all sense of who I was, then bounced back to a more normal way of being, although the diminution of identity remained permanent, even as it shifted into more of a background state.

The last story in this section describes how motivations can change after awakening:

When I lost my Core Veil, it was pretty subtle, so I wasn't sure it had happened, although I knew something had happened because somehow the sky just felt more open in some soft way. During the next month, I felt pretty much unmotivated to do anything. I spent most of the time lying on my bed. I knew something was different, but I didn't know what it was. I asked myself if I was depressed, and I wasn't. I noticed that when I would consider doing something, like go to a gathering or function, I literally didn't see any difference in going or not going, and since I was already where I was, it was easier to just stay home. This changed at some point (I do enjoy gatherings) but what I realized was that the 'juice' that had been feeding my motivation to do things was mostly ego-based, and now much of that juice wasn't there. As time passed, I began to do things, pretty much as before, but I was not doing them from a position of how I would show up, or what I would get out of a situation. I did things just for the sake of doing them, more out of curiosity, to see what would happen, without a vested interest in the outcome. This was a huge relief for me, and continues to be, and allows me to enjoy life in a way I never had previously, and notice things more as they are than how I think they should be. Outwardly, nothing really changed much, and I don't think others noticed much change in me. It was not dramatic, but in a subtle and profound way I see things completely differently than before and I am more available to be with things as they are.

This experience of lost motivation does happen occasionally after awakening, since our motivations are ego-based and a core sense of ego has just been lost. If this occurs, there will be a time factor, which will vary from person to person, before the integration completes and allows motivation to arise from a new place. This story also nicely illuminates how after basic awakening, everything changes and yet everything remains the same.

The Journey

From the beginning of your incarnational journey, you have been experiencing yourself as a particular separate being. You accumulated a treasure trove of experiences, all of which deepened your identity as this separate being. You developed issues and accumulated karma knots, which continued to deepen your sense of separateness, and with that your experience of struggle and suffering. When you got as deep into this constructed illusion as you could, when there was nowhere else for you to go, something turned inside. Instead of accumulating identities and issues, you began to shed them. Slowly, very slowly, you were now journeying back to the light, to the reality of what you truly are. At some point—perhaps first in this life—you came across the idea of inner freedom, and something in you recognized what that was and began to move towards it. If the pull was deep enough, your journey accelerated.

At some point, the idea of spiritual awakening—which is the breaking down of the Core Veil—entered your reality. At the present time, this may still just be an interesting idea for you, or it may have become something that strongly pulls on your heart. In either case, I can tell you with certainty that if you have reached the point where a book about something as deeply rooted in Divinity as VortexHealing has come into your hands, then awakening is possible for you in this life.

There are many paths to awakening. Some of them will awaken you in this lifetime and some won't. The fastest path to basic awakening that I know of is through the VortexHealing lineage. Divine intention for the VortexHealing lineage is to facilitate spiritual awakening, so the divine Source of the lineage generates the 'ripening' that is needed for this, and then provides classes in which awakening is generated *for all the students in the class*. Yet VortexHealing is not for everyone. If it is for you, you will either feel drawn to it, or something in you will simply know that this is where you need to go.

There is a deep irony embedded within our spiritual journey. Although our experience is that it is our personal, separate self that is seeking freedom, it is only because Divinity is calling us home that we are seeking it. In addition, because we experience ourselves as having started this journey, we believe we will be there at the end of it. But at the end of the journey, there is no more seeker; there is just our own true nature, which is the One that was calling us home.

What Awakening Means for Healing Issues

On a body level, awakening creates a huge acceleration in the energy system, making it much more fluid. This makes it easier to heal body conditions, and it promotes longevity.

The larger impact, though, is for emotional issues. All emotional issues are rooted in the egoic sense of a personal self that has to struggle to survive and feel safe. As long as that is one's core identity, that drama must continue to play out in some way. Therapy and healing can do a lot to soften the edges of that drama, to lower our reactivity, to enable us to cope better, to make us healthier, to help us feel more relaxed in our lives, and to help our lives be more enjoyable and satisfying. Therapy and healing can improve our lives in many ways, but without awakening, the core experience that runs through every moment of our life cannot be transformed. No matter how good life gets, that sense of a personal self that is struggling and feels threatened will continue. Even if the places where we struggle and suffer are pushed to the background, they will always be the center around which everything else in our life revolves. Since all emotional issues are based on this separateness, it becomes very difficult to finish with an issue, as its fundamental cause will still be in place. With awakening, that all changes, and a new freedom in relation to all our issues takes root in our psyche and hearts.

What Awakening Means for Practicing VortexHealing®

The kind of healing tools that can be given to someone who has lost their Core Veil is of a very different order than what can be given to someone who hasn't had this kind of awakening. There are two reasons for this: the huge evolution in the person's energy system enables a much higher level of divine transmission to be integrated into it, and the person's awareness now bridges deeper into creation. Because of the way healing transmissions work, healing tools that will work at higher dimensional levels—for instance, to clear higher dimensional blueprints and conditioning—need the healer to have awakened to that level. The awakeness at that level makes it possible for the healer to channel, by intention, healing tools that function at that level.

For other energy healing systems, since spiritual awakening is not part of the agenda, they can never teach healing tools that rise to that level. Yet those who continue with VortexHealing classes through to awakening are in a different situation. The shift in consciousness and the evolution in the energy system created by the awakening enable higher-level VortexHealing transmissions to be given that are truly astounding.

A taste of the depth of what is possible with the Grace available through VortexHealing can show up in healing sessions in interesting ways. One student shared this story:

> She told me that her aunt, who is a nurse, said she wanted to try VortexHealing. It was her first experience with energy healing, and she was nervous. The aunt said afterwards she saw lots of light and colors and felt waves of energy moving through her. Two days later, the student asked her if God or angels had ever appeared for her. The aunt said that twice in her life, in times of crisis, she had prayed for help and God has appeared as a light. Both times the experiences were very moving and transformative. "That's how I knew the healing you did was real," the aunt told her. "It was the third time I experienced God."

Embodiment

"Embodiment" is the word we often use for learning to live from our awakening. Imagine that your consciousness is like a sea of movement that covers a deeper level of your being. You don't notice that deeper place because you have become entranced with that movement, so that is all you see. Awakening creates a spot of stillness within all that movement. When your awareness is in that stillness, you lose the distraction of the movement and your deeper being makes itself known.

However, even after the awakening, there is still so much movement around that spot, and you are still entranced enough with it, that your attention tends to go back to the movement. Embodiment is the process by which you learn to keep more of your attention out of that movement and in your deeper being. As you do so, the resting in your inner being quiets more of the movement. The spot of stillness then grows larger, and it becomes easier to keep your awareness there, enabling you to more easily live and act from your deeper being. Without embodiment, although the awakening is still there, it tends to move further and further into the background of your consciousness, and then you mostly live from the movement on the surface, which is not what you really are.

Another analogy is that of awakening from a very deep and very intense dream. When you first wake up, your consciousness is still full of the dream. As you rest there, awake, you can allow yourself to be pulled back into the dream—more like a daydream now, since you are awake—or you can let go of the dream and focus on bringing yourself more into awakeness. The latter is like embodiment. It is moving more of your awareness into what is awake, so you can live and act from there.

Here is a student's comment about her embodiment process:

> *The more I have embodied and deepened within my awakening, I have noticed I've become less reactive to the way I respond to my conditioning. In my experience, the awakening process has awakened me out of conditioning and awakened me into the truth of who I am, that which is ever-present pure love & Divinity itself. Losing my Core Veil was*

not a big deal to me in the moment. However as I continued
with the awakening classes, I noticed I was ripening, and it
was through this ripening that I was able to recognize how I
have deepened and embodied.

Awakenings are like vertical movements. Each one creates a *deeper* opening within you. Yet to really have the full experience of that awakening, you have to live it; you have to embody it. That is a horizontal movement. With embodiment, your awakening gets *wider*.

Most of your embodiment, by its very nature, cannot be done in a class; it needs to be done on an ongoing basis, day to day, since this is about how you are living your life—how you are living your awakening. However, to support this ongoing process, VortexHealing provides embodiment classes. For many students, their most profound experiences of awakening happen in these embodiment classes. (We currently call these classes *Opening to Oneness & Divinity.*)

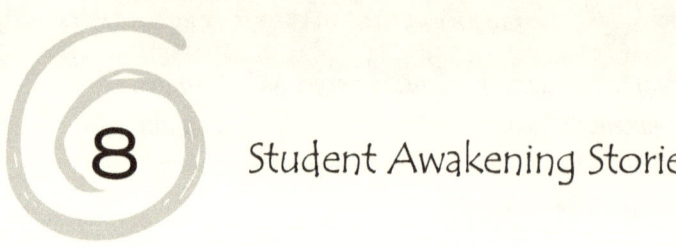

8 Student Awakening Stories

Because we experience life through the lens of separateness, there is always a gap between ourselves and everything else. The rest of life becomes an object in our consciousness, so we lose a sense of direct connection with it. This makes the rest of life seem less than fully real, and our lives lose that richness we had as a child and become flat. We crave intense experiences to compensate for this, but even those are lived from within the bubble of our separateness and so don't fulfill us. We are still stuck within our bubble of separateness, continuously self-referencing ourselves, as we endlessly replay and talk to ourselves about our life experiences with nonstop stories in our minds. No matter how much we try to engage life, our life experience is played out more in the separate mind-bubble in our heads than in our hearts. Our experience becomes a sort of instant replay with commentary, rather than the richness and wholeness that we seek.

In the awakening stories shared by students below, you'll find a large continuum of different experiences. They range from surprise, to the confusion that can arise when the sense of 'I' disappears, to the joy and peace and spaciousness that is available when the bubble of separateness bursts and life flows through. As you read these stories, my hope is that it will give you a momentary taste of what is beyond your own bubble.

Some of the stories refer to basic awakening and some refer to later awakenings.

Attending the recent BodyMind Awakening class is the most profound change for me of all the classes. I feel joyful and aliveness and love daily since taking the class. Words feel inadequate to describe the changes. Heartfelt gratitude.

Losing the Core Veil was like getting rid of a too small, too tight piece of clothing. Coming home, I always felt closer to the trees; they looked to me more green, and bright. Later the 'I' was just an empty echo in the head, not in the heart. The 'life movie' gets easier.

I want to say that the 7-day Embodiment class is now one of my favorites ever. I think the best way to describe what it did for me is that it fundamentally changed my experience of myself from being a person experiencing Awakeness, to that of Awakeness experiencing this person. It's a big difference! In addition, my psychic vision is much, much better, I feel like I have a positive, friendly relationship with the whole universe, and I really enjoy having a place to go and rest - quiet emptiness - whenever I need it.

After awakening to 0-self [a certain level of awakening], my nervous system was in shock for a while as I had lost a sense of navigation that depended on self and other. It was as if I could no longer get a grip on anything and for months my vision would try its hardest to grip on what it saw as other and couldn't. It was quite unsettling and this continued for months before settling down, as if the one looking for other just eventually ran out of steam. Then it just relaxed into what is.

During one of the awakening classes, I was sitting in a bus in London, upstairs. I was looking through the window. This was such an amazing "experience" for me. I looked through the window of the bus, and there were no people on the street. There was (and still is) only the ONE movement of LIFE itself.

For me, a lot of absolutely crazy fear came up to the surface. My mind was going bonkers trying to find that familiar sense of 'I' in my system. My whole life I was so deeply in survival that I made myself believe there was no survival energy in my life. I was always incredibly brave, and needed to accomplish so much that fear was not an option, so I made myself believe there was no fear. Haha... was I ever in for a big surprise....

Many years ago I hurt my foot while training in a gym and I needed to go to work the next day. So I took two Solpadine, which is a painkiller and contains codeine. Not only was my foot in less pain but I felt the edge was taken off the day. So the second day I took two more, and because my foot was in less pain the second day, I noticed even more how the edge was gone from the day. When I say "edge" I mean some kind of harshness, if you can understand that. So I noticed after my second awakening class that this edge or harshness was gone from my life and has never come back. A lot of women in Ireland are addicted to codeine products and now I know why. And all they need is self-realization—cheaper in the long run and better for them.

Just got back from BodyMind Awakening class last night. After a good night sleep and a lazy start of the day I took a walk, no longer being in a group or group field, completely on my own, being able to let it sink in and feel what happened. There was (is) soooooooo much awareness in my body, no boundaries between the awareness inside my body and the awareness surrounding it. Felt like awareness was walking within itself. The stillness and the beauty of it moved me to tears. Still can't believe what has happened to me.

On losing the Inner Veil, the experience was of seeing myself as pure awareness, and as I looked out I saw awareness looking back at me from every direction. It was eternal beingness.

Wasn't so sure how I felt about day one [of Core Veil class], even though everyone's Core Veil got released. Couldn't really track the release, which was a surprise, although I did track the veil thinning over the course of the day. And, although I could feel a new spaciousness in the heart and an overall energetic softness, in other respects I didn't feel much of a difference.

However, it turns out the loss of the Core Veil was just a teeing up for the second day. We started by releasing the "I-thought" veil aspect [a secondary veil created by the Core Veil]. THAT was HUGE for me. Suddenly the new spaciousness, which felt mostly restricted to the heart, moved up into the head. It was what I had thought losing the Core Veil would be like. Like being in a beautiful space of peace from a meditation, if I actually meditated.

We released a few more veil aspects individually, much more quickly than in classes past, each one of which was huge. Ric then moved ALL the rest AT ONCE, in about 20 minutes, which had never previously been done in a class. And that was just before lunch. Epic, and beyond description!!

Before Core Veil I had always attracted very dominant, aggressive aloof men. My relationships were always short, like a few months to a year. Now I'm happy that I could finish the chapter of bad relationships and enter the chapter of a real loving relationship. This is my awakening experience: I could enter love, light, and peace!

I went to the gym today and the most incredible thing happened. It was like I remembered how to do things I had never been able to do before— at least since I got sick when I was 18. I was able to move, bend, run, and lift in a way I have never been able to before. I was automatically completing yoga poses that I have only seen others do. I have taken maybe eight yoga classes in my life! I would start a class and then drop it quickly as it hurt too much to continue. I'm not hurting now. My jaw and head are still a little tight but the rest of my body feels entirely different! I'm accomplishing twice as much in half the time physically.

This is seriously blowing my mind! I had to tell you. I had to tell somebody. I'm grateful for what ever is happening. I just don't quite understand it.

To think such things could result from a shift in perspective [from an awakening] is almost impossible for me to imagine. Even if it was a really big one.

And my balance was amazing! I've been faking good balance for 22 years. Yes, it is possible to fake it. Fancying myself a dancer before I got ill, it was really hard on me to lose the ability to move the way I had before, so I created an illusion of balance and flexibility. What ever is happening now is the real thing. My nerve pathways can't have just regenerated just like that. Something else must be happening.

I want to add that the body stuff isn't the only interesting thing happening. I feel like my language system finally works. I'm no longer a non-linear girl trying desperately to live in a linear world. Everything fits now. For the first time in my life I'm not terrified of getting up in the morning or walking down the street. It's strange, I know, to say I felt terrified all the time before and now I'm not. But it's the truth.

At that point [of awakening] my whole being felt like it dropped. Gave way. My neck muscles gave out, and my whole body went into a deep relaxation. It felt like time had stopped. Momentarily groggy, heavy. Like

I had woken from an anesthesia. I looked up at the trees, heard the birds sing their sunset songs and then looked down at my own body. I touched my arms to feel if all of this was real.... There, at that moment, there was just being.

There are no words to describe the awakening, because it is life itself succeeding every moment. It's like water running through the water. It is the same Grace filling with love everything that was, is, and will be.

With my first awakening, when losing the Core Veil, I felt a sense of letting go into the unknown, and with it came this deep peaceful love that was endless, like an ocean of peaceful love.

When I first learned about VortexHealing, I already had a deep desire to get to the other side of my intense suffering – I had the motivation, I just needed the right tools to get me there. VortexHealing provided me with the tools I needed to accelerate my process and evolution in ways I never thought possible. Today, any suffering I feel is largely overshadowed by the clarity and Freedom that has become a permanent part of my experience. I cannot recommend this path enough!

Losing my Core Veil was one of the most profound moments of my life. It was in the first awakening classes, before Ric was able to pop all the Core Veils at once, so people repeated the class until their Core Veil popped. It was such a powerful movement of Grace! I loved watching how Ric would take each person who was ripe and ready into the popping of their Core Veil moment. As we sat doing meditations to help release whatever was holding us back from 'popping' the Core Veil, I suddenly realized that I was so attached to the divine that I couldn't become one with the divine, which made me laugh at myself for hours. When I spoke to Ric, he pulled out a coin and holding it in front of me said: "Blow your attachment to the divine into this coin." Upon doing so I felt lighter, and then as he did a coin trick and made the coin disappear, my Core Veil popped! My heart started spinning in what felt like three directions at once and I felt myself being in the whole cosmos and all the dimensions at once. When I spoke my voice sounded like it was someone else's and was no longer coming from what I had previously believed to be 'me'. It seemed to be coming from the oneness of everything. That night I cried, realizing that everything up to date had in fact been an illusion, and a new reality was occurring. I laughed more than I ever laughed before at the cosmic joke of life. I can only describe it as a birth into a new reality of love and pure truth. Amazing!

It has been very interesting for me to look what has changed or is changing since basic awakening. For me it is like a permanent connection to the divine, so much inner peace and freedom. It's like to be in a permanent inner flow - living my life from my heart - and everything follows this flow and works the best for me. There is already the well-known inner struggle but it doesn't touch me like before. My life feels like adoring the divine all the time. I can feel the love of all creation - which I never felt before. When I first felt Vortex energy in my body I knew that this would be my path, like coming home.

After the Inner Veil awakening class, I have achieved a lasting stillness that permeates through my entire life and all my relationships. It is like there is space within me, and when conditioned reactions arise I can see them for what they are, rather than letting them become me. The result is a life lived with far more freedom and a joy in everything that I see or do. Beforehand, I was in the prison of my conceptual mind and its story. I have started living life.

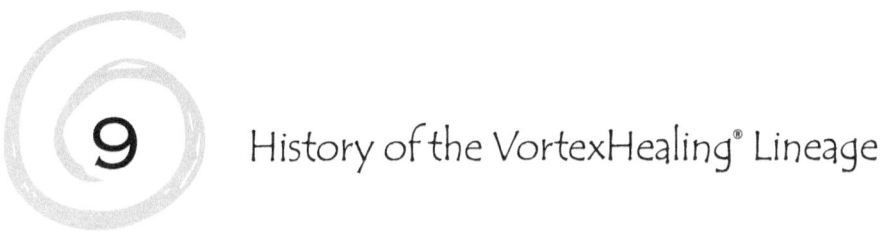

9   History of the VortexHealing® Lineage

My Story

I had been working with various healing modalities for over 15 years. It was November 26, 1994, and I was visiting my mother in Douglaston, New York. I stood in the center of the room that I was about to sleep in, and I started to clear the energy of the room.

When I first started to clear spaces, I would sit in the middle of the space and expand my energy field into the space, using the energy to push out the build up of negative energy. This was slow and not very efficient. Yet earlier that year, I had discovered that I somehow knew how to access a very unique energy. This energy was white, very sparkly, very active, and easily directed by my own intent. I could just pull it out of somewhere—I didn't know where exactly—with my hands, and intend it to do something, like clean a room, or even the whole house, and it did so in less than a minute, leaving the space clear, fresh, and sparkling with light. I sensed I learned how to do this in a past life.

So, that evening in my mother's house, I stood in the middle of the room I was to sleep in and reached into creation to pull out this newly discovered energy. But when I pulled, I somehow also pulled open a sort of trap door in the universe—as if the energy had been attached to it—and suddenly I was standing in the middle of an enormous Vortex, in some other dimension, with my feet somehow still on the ground. As I tried to understand what was happening, a voice began to speak to me out of this Vortex.

The voice called itself Merlin. I was told that I had used this Vortex in the past, in two lives in England, and it was time to use it again. I could heal with it, but first I had to reacquaint myself with it. I soon began to use this Vortex in my healing practice with some amazing results. Some of those early healing stories were shared earlier, in *Chapter 2: How Effective is VortexHealing®?*

Through those early healings, I had come to realize that VortexHealing was the most powerful healing art I had ever encountered. Yet I had no thought to teach it. I couldn't even explain how I did it myself—somehow my energy system just did it when I intended it to—it still had the past life knowledge. However, after enough requests from people wanting to learn it, I asked Merlin if I could. The answer was a strong affirmative, and that it would take five days. I was more than a little doubtful. I couldn't imagine how it would be possible to teach something at that level in just five days, especially when I didn't even know how I was doing it myself.

The first class was given in Tucson, Arizona, September 2, 1995, about nine months after my own initial experience. When class started, I still had my doubts as to how well this was going to work. I hadn't realized yet that I wasn't really the one teaching it. Merlin was the one in charge, teaching VortexHealing by direct consciousness transmission. He was the one accelerating their energy systems to get them ready to receive the transmission, and he was the one giving them the healing tools. My job was simply to show up, make my energy field available for the transmission, and explain to everyone what was happening.

To my surprise, by the fourth day, everyone was able to easily channel VortexHealing's divine energy and consciousness. From there, it has grown into what it is today.

The History of the Lineage

The VortexHealing lineage began with a man named Mehindra who lived about 5600 years ago. Mehindra was not a typical 'karmic' human being—he was not a soul or incarnational personality. He was an avatar—a divine expression incarnated into a human body. Every avatar brings a unique aspect of divine expression into manifestation. The aspect of Divinity that Mehindra manifests is transformational magic.

However, VortexHealing didn't come into being until thousands of years later. In 753 B.C., a man living in what is now England, who was close to awakening, received the gift of VortexHealing as a divine revelation.

In his vision, Mehindra presented himself as 'Merlin', a name chosen because it was the closest word vibrationally in the language of that area to the quality of transformational magic. Working with this divine gift, the man awakened and began to pass the gift on to others, through the mechanism of direct consciousness transmission. This was the beginning of the Merlin lineage on Earth and the beginning of VortexHealing.

Along the way, the lineage was 'lost' and re-discovered several times. The Merlin of myth was actually the fifth Merlin of the lineage. The name "Merlin" was a title, given to a teacher of the lineage who had reached a certain level of oneness with the Merlin that is the divine Source of our lineage. There were quite a few VortexHealing teachers who never became a Merlin.

The lineage was recovered in modern times by myself, in November 1994, as described earlier. I became the 13th Merlin of the lineage, as well as its "lineage holder". Because of the nature of the acceleration of awakening today, both within this lineage and in humanity as a whole, anyone capable of becoming a VortexHealing teacher today would also have reached the level of being a Merlin.

As lineage holder, I have passed on the VortexHealing teacher transmission to others, who now teach VortexHealing in various parts of the world. Yet the spread of VortexHealing worldwide is not its most fundamental change since I first recovered it, in 1994. Rather, it is the enormous evolution that VortexHealing itself has undergone since then. The depth and power of it today is indeed remarkable. When you experience what VortexHealing is able to do, you will know why the name Merlin is so associated with magic.

VortexHealing entered a new phase when Merlin facilitated my spiritual awakening in August 2002. Classes were soon developed to facilitate this awakening for students as well. As these classes progressed and deepened, it became clear that Merlin's divine intention was for all students of his lineage to be awakened. VortexHealing now has two interweaving manifestations: that of a healing art and that of an awakening path. At a certain level of training now, any student can take the class that dissolves the Core Veil, the center of the ego-structure in the human personality, moving them into spiritual awakening.

VortexHealing is presently taught around the world by the certified teachers shown on the home page of VortexHealing website (*www. vortexhealing.org*).

The Play of the Divine

Throughout this book, I have written that VortexHealing is a divine lineage that is being manifested by divine intention and guided by divine intelligence. It would be easy for a reader to take such statements as general concepts and not consider the true significance of this. However, what these concepts mean in concrete terms is that when you channel the VortexHealing tools, the divine, avataric presence we call Merlin is actually present with you. It is present in what you are channeling and it is present with you in your field. In addition, it is available for both meditation and personal guidance.

Over time, that guidance has become very obvious to me— concretely obvious. Although much of the divine guidance I receive is subtle and in the background, in my role as lineage holder, sometimes I need that guidance to be in my face. Without that, the discovery of new VortexHealing tools would be a haphazard process. Yet Merlin guides me to them in direct and very obvious ways. The sum of that guidance becomes the continuously evolving history of the lineage.

The simplest example of this occurred while I was teaching a class in Israel. As I was talking to students, suddenly a large ball of light appeared in front of my face that blocked my vision somewhat. It stayed for several minutes. It was clearly from Merlin, and it only disappeared when I communicated to him that I would explore what this was after class. That night, in meditation, I received that ball of light into my energy system and discovered that it was the transmission for our next level of healing tool. I hadn't been looking for this healing tool. Yet divine intention, aware of the bigger picture, both knew it was time for this to be manifested and *arranged* for it to be manifested in a way that was impossible for me to miss.

It is very endearing to have the divine 'play' with you in this way. Not only do you get the message, but you start to recognize that the idea that Divinity is with you and guiding you is much more than an idea. Recognizing the reality of this in your day-to-day existence is its own kind of awakening, which changes everything in your life. Divinity is then experienced, on a human level, as a friend that is continuously playing with you as it guides you home.

I'll share one more example that illuminates just how perfect this 'play of the Divine' can be and how much power is available to Divinity to manipulate events as needed. I was on my way to teach a VortexHealing class in Cork, Ireland, in September 1998, and things immediately started to go wrong involving time and timing. First, as I was checking in for my flight, I was told that my second flight had been canceled and I had to be rerouted. Next, I actually got onto the wrong plane. The ticket agent had looked at my ticket, of course, but she wasn't supposed to see that it was the wrong ticket, so she didn't. It was only when an announcement about the flight came over the airplane speakers that I realized I was on the wrong plane. Luckily, it hadn't taken off yet.

This was just the warm-up. I almost lost my jacket in the next airport, and by the time I got to Ireland, I realized that my watch had broken. By then, I expected that my luggage would not be there when I went to collect it, and it wasn't. When my luggage did eventually arrive, my alarm clock, which had been fine the last time I had used it, was now broken. I now had the conscious idea that there was something odd going on with me in relation to timing and time.

In class the next morning, I shared what was happening to me and told the class that "it was as if my timeline had been broken." Merlin had managed by now to get the concept of a broken timeline active enough in my mind that I was communicating it to others, even though I still didn't really know what the concept meant. However, Merlin was still reinforcing his point—he was still *playing* with me about time—so when I bought a replacement watch to have one for the class, within a few days it was broken as well.

I recognized that I was in the middle of receiving some kind of divine teaching, but at this point I didn't realize that all of these events were just the setup, the preparation, so I would have the concept of a 'broken timeline' in my mind when the actual breaking of a timeline occurred.

Merlin scheduled that (without my knowing of course) for the end of the last day of class.

I was on my way to meet Anthony Gorman, another VortexHealing teacher. I was crossing the street in the middle of a sharp curve in Cork, where traffic merges from several directions. I was used to traffic moving in the opposite way in America, and it made that corner all the more confusing, which was part of the setup, of course. I was almost across the street when I heard the screeching of the brakes of a bus, just inches from me. In that moment, it was as if time stopped, and something in my energy field rippled out in a funny kind of expansion, then rippled back, and I thought, "Oh, almost died." I could feel the bus driver cursing at me, but I just kept walking. I found Anthony, got into his car, and as I told him what had happened, he immediately noticed that I actually looked very different, that the right side of my body had lost a significant amount of dense conditioning. In fact it was so much lighter that when I met my wife, Susanne, a few days later, she was actually shocked at how much my system had changed. Yet as I sat there with Anthony, it was quite clear what had happened, since Merlin had prepared me to know this: my timeline had been broken, and the effect was a very deep, virtually instantaneous healing. Thankfully, Merlin had made sure, so precisely sure, that not only did I have the concept of a broken timeline active in my mind then, but that the bus driver who was to facilitate the movement was actually paying attention as he came around that curve, or it would have been my head and bones broken instead of my timeline.

Yet Merlin hadn't set all these events in motion just to do a healing on me. Rather, he was teaching me about a new kind of healing that could be done with divine energy and consciousness, called "Breaking Timelines". So when I got home, as an added touch of divine play and to keep what had happened fresh in my consciousness, I found that a cute little clock I had bought in Ireland had now stopped working as well. All I could do was laugh. Soon after, Merlin showed me how to use his divine energy and consciousness to intentionally break a timeline for healing, and he created a new transmission for this so that students could learn to break timelines in their healing sessions as well.

These events were a manifestation of divine guidance for the

VortexHealing lineage. In fact, the history of the lineage is the history of events such as these. Yet this is how all of your own personal histories get formed as well: by divine intention and intelligence guiding you and bringing appropriate events into your lives. Usually you don't notice, because most of it is subtler than the examples I have given here, and some of it is painful. Yet the fact of it remains, and you only need to notice it once to know that it is happening always. Divinity is always with you, here and now. Knowing this and opening to the sense of it will change your life forever.

10   VortexHealing® Classes

When I first recovered VortexHealing, I had no intention of teaching it. I didn't even think it was possible for me to do so. However, people were noticing the amazing healings it created and kept asking if I could teach it to them. Eventually, I did. And from that one Basic/Foundational class it has grown into all the different levels of classes that are offered, worldwide, today.

VortexHealing now offers two distinct but interconnected paths of classes: a healing path and an awakening path. They are interconnected because our deepest healing classes require spiritual awakening as a pre-requisite. The five-day Basic/Foundational training needs to be taken before any of the other VortexHealing classes can be taken. No previous experience in energy healing is required.

The classes are organized into five levels of pre-awakening classes and two 'threads' of post-awakening classes, with one of those threads being a healing thread and the other being a thread for deeper awakening classes.

Throughout all the early classes, there is a 'ripening towards awakening' reflected in the rapid loss of karma knots. As I wrote earlier, all karma knots are gone by the end of the third class. This is just the beginning. As the ripening continues, the divine Source of the lineage ensures that by the time the prerequisites for an awakening class have been taken, all students are ripe enough for that to occur. In the *Core Veil and Awakening to Being Awareness* class, losing the Core Veil is the agenda for the first day.

The divine Source of our lineage has set it up so that students can be taken through an ongoing awakening process, level by level. In our 'awakening thread' of classes, each class takes students through the specific awakening movements that they have become ripe for, from previous classes. If an understanding of these levels interests you, you can read through the class descriptions on the VortexHealing website, *(www.vortexhealing.org)*, or you can find the awakening map we use in my book, *Awakening Through the Veils.*

The healing tools, the deep transformations that happen in trainings, and the awakening movements are not generated by the teachers of the trainings but by the divine presence that operates through them, which is the source of the classes and our lineage. The healing tools are given by 'direct consciousness transmission', transmitted directly from divine consciousness to the student's consciousness and energy system. The awakenings are created in a similar manner, directly from the divine Source of the lineage.

On the VortexHealing website, are all the details you might want to know about the classes offered: worldwide schedule, class prices, what is taught in each class, the prerequisite for each class, and organizer contact information. For more details or to register for a class, you'd call or email the organizer listed for that class. In some non-English speaking countries, some classes are taught in English and translated, and some are taught in the native language.

Although VortexHealing offers a comprehensive program in healing and awakening, the Basic/Foundational class is a complete energy healing art. No previous experience is necessary, and you can take this class without any commitment to do other ones. From this one class, you will gain a magnificent healing tool that you can use on yourself or others, in-person or at a distance, for the rest of your life.

The one thing you can most count on from taking a VortexHealing class is that it will evolve your energy system and have a transformative effect on your life.

Here is one student's story:

When I felt Vortex energy in my body for the first time, I knew that that would be my path. It's difficult to describe how fulfilling it is, to use Vortex energy on myself or on others. It's great to feel the energy of Vortex every day, to discover my issues and to uncover my clients' issues. To sit in the energy while channeling is like coming home to feel pure love and pure magic. It's wonderful to be able to get in such depth. Since I started to practice VortexHealing, I'm full of energy and I feel so much more grounded. I never had had this feeling before. To discover my true source and be in permanent contact with it is indescribable. Sometimes I think about a goal and a very short time later it is fulfilled - incredible! Every day is full of joy and there is a deep feeling that everything will develop in the right way. I live my life from my inner source always knowing what to do. With clients there is a deep connection, and there is a huge amount of grace and thankfulness. To practice VortexHealing is the biggest luck of my life. Merlin and the Divine are the best attendants for my ongoing transformation and my whole life. While I'm writing this I can feel a huge energy in my body - there is a connection to the whole universe. I feel so grateful!

11   A Magical Path

As you have seen, VortexHealing is a very effective healing art. However, in describing what VortexHealing is, what it can do, and how it works, what gets lost is the pure magic of this healing art and the joy that comes from practicing it.

When you are using VortexHealing on yourself or someone else, you are not simply an empty channel through which healing is happening. You are an active part of that process. First of all, you feel all the magical energy and divine presence that is coming through you, and it feels wonderful. In fact, just experiencing that on a regular basis is a transformative process that aligns you with a deeper sense of inner joy and freedom. In addition, you get to direct where all this lovely energy is being focused, so there is the experience of playing with divine magic and watching it have magical effects in the receiver. This is a profound creative process that is deeply enjoyable. The excitement it generates comes through pretty clearly in many of the student stories shared in this book. In addition, when the receiver is a friend, family member, or a client, they love what they experience through your healing, and you get to share that with them. When the receiver is yourself, not only do you get to enjoy the results of the healing, but through ongoing self-healings you enter into a new phase of self-discovery, as the healings illuminate your inner process. You learn about your emotional patterns, your mental attitudes, your attachments and avoidances, and how all that plays out through your body and energy system.

When you practice VortexHealing, in addition to whatever healing occurs, you engage your creativity, deepen self-awareness, and have a joyful and magically transformative experience. Yet there is more: practicing VortexHealing simultaneously deepens your connection with Divinity, transforms you with divine love, and brings you to awakening, breaking down your bubble of separateness and opening you to the inner freedom that is your own true nature.

Everyone is on a path that will eventually return them to the Divinity from whence they came. No matter what path you choose, you will eventually end up in the same place. So ultimately, it is about the journey, and you have the freedom to choose your path. VortexHealing is the magical path. It invites you to play with Divinity and divine magic as you make your way home.

Here is one student's story:

> I have been searching for something like VortexHealing from a very young age. I'm a bit of a reader; anything to do with magic appealed to me. Later this changed into reading all sorts of books about spiritual development and spiritual awakening. In the end, I found VortexHealing—or did VortexHealing find me?
>
> I had been working as a holistic physical therapist for about 15 years. Although I really liked my work, I was also looking for something that could take it a good step further. Something that would be a structural asset to it. Not another class or another technique, useful as they can be. In the meantime, I was also looking for someone who could help my son, who is autistic. The psychiatrist said there was nothing she could do to help him. She made a diagnosis, and that was it. I didn't believe her. So I started looking around to see if I could find someone who could help my son.
>
> One day I was sitting in a flower remedies course and the lady who taught it had a table full of books and leaflets on the Bach Flower Remedies. But there was also a blue leaflet lying there that was different. My eye fell on one word: MERLIN. As my son's name is Arthur and I have a passion for Celtic history, I have read a lot of books about those two. So I picked up the leaflet and skimmed through it.
>
> To make a long story short, after only four sessions of VortexHealing my son improved dramatically. He was so

much more relaxed, open, cuddly, grounded, and cheerful. It was a truly amazing change. And the changes were permanent. After a while I realized that this VortexHealing was maybe something for me as well. After one or two sessions with the practitioner, he told me I could take classes to learn this, and to my surprise, there was a class in a town less than an hour's drive from where I live.

So I enrolled in the Basic/Foundational course, being very critical, despite the wonderful transformation of my son. I could hear myself thinking: I'm not going to listen to any spiritual nonsense. If I don't like this, I will be out of here in no time!

Well, I am still doing VortexHealing classes, and I have been doing VortexHealing on clients from that class onwards, as this so beautifully compliments my work as a holistic physical therapist. I have found exactly what I was looking for.

VortexHealing opens up a completely new dimension for me. As if I have been walking along a wall trying to find a gate to the other side and finally find it. And it surpasses every expectation! In addition to the fact that many of my clients are very enthusiastic and helped by it, VortexHealing supports a growing insight for me into how people develop all sorts of mental, emotional, and physical issues/complaints, and it gives me a deep understanding of how that impacts their lives. This understanding helps me to open up to them in a very compassionate way. And as I open up to the Divinity coming through me, I can let intuitions materialize that help people along. I can be a vehicle to make things more conscious for them.

But most of all, VortexHealing has helped me to live from Divinity, so I just do what I can in an attentive, compassionate, and loving way, however small the situation. I can now open up to be an increasingly available instrument of Divine love and light. I'm learning to be selfless, while still taking care of myself, since I still have my own struggles, problems, and issues, and a body that sometimes aches. I'm grateful to have VortexHealing, which I use to improve so many things, like better sleep, more energy, less attachments, being able to let go, etc.

Being able to create a healing for someone else or myself, just by intending and channeling VortexHealing, is the purest magic to me. From oneness, this magic is brought into a human being, and something gets healed. All of this gives me space and freedom and joy. And it gives me a very deep sense of inner peace. Coping with living in this world has changed enormously for me.

I'm grateful every day that I came across VortexHealing. It has made life so much better and fuller, quieter inside, and surprisingly, much more grounded.

Stories like this are not untypical among VortexHealers. Beginning with the Basic/Foundational class, whatever their initial motivations were for taking the class, their lives transform. How could they not transform when they are engaged so actively with Divinity? VortexHealing was designed to create transformation. In addition to being an amazing healing art, it is a magical path.

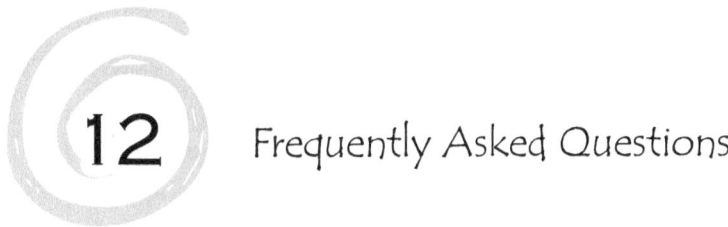

1. Since VortexHealing can be used as a spiritual path, do I need to give up other paths, teachers or practices when I take VortexHealing classes? Not at all. VortexHealing is universal. It will support you on whatever path you are on and with any other teachers you are drawn to. In addition, it finds no conflict in simultaneously working with other healing or spiritual practices. VortexHealing is an 'open' path; there is nothing in your life that you need to change to participate in it.

2. Does Channeling VortexHealing drain your personal energy? No, it doesn't, because the practitioner is not using their own personal energy. They are only acting as a conduit, using divine energy and consciousness. However, since the process brings divine energy and consciousness through their personal energy field, this kind of channeling is typically both energizing for the channeler and has a long-term transformational effect. In addition, just as exercise evolves the physical conditioning of the body, this kind of channeling is like energetic exercise, and it evolves and strengthens the practitioner's energy system.

3. How do I try out a VortexHealing session? On the VortexHealing website, *www.vortexhealing.org*, there is a button that says. "Find A Healer". If you click on it, you will be taken to a page with a drop-down menu of countries. When you pick your country, you get a list of healers with phone numbers, and the list shows you what level of VortexHealing each person has taken. A student needs to have done five courses before they can join the list. In general I suggest getting sessions from students with the highest levels of training. Since VortexHealing works very well at a distance, where you live is not a factor for getting a session.

4. Can VortexHealing be used on animals? Yes, VortexHealing can be used on animals, in person or at a distance. It can be used on any living creature or plant. As demonstrated earlier, it can also be used on non-living things, such musical instruments. And it can be used to transform the energy of living spaces, work spaces, or even towns and cities.

5. Can VortexHealing be done on a group of people? Yes, but at least the second class, Magical Structures, needs to be taken for a practitioner to be able to do group healing. The group can be in person or at a distance.

6. Does doing VortexHealing on others also heal the healer? It does and it doesn't. While you are channeling VortexHealing, you are in a state of resonating with Divinity, as all that divine energy and consciousness comes through you. This evolves your energy system, raises your vibrational frequency, and purifies your consciousness. As a result, there is a general movement towards greater health and well-being. Yet what you are channeling is going to the other person, not to yourself. The focus of divine intention for healing is on the receiver. Yet you still receive the indirect benefits that come from being aligned with and a vehicle for divine energy and consciousness. In addition, there is the simple joy of channeling this magical divine energy, which opens the heart.

7. VortexHealing keeps evolving the healing transmissions in its classes. Do I need to repeat the classes to get the "upgraded" versions? When healing transmissions are upgraded, that upgrade goes out to everyone who has ever taken that class. There has only ever been one upgrade, at the highest level of VortexHealing, that couldn't be given at a distance. It was a massive upgrade—a completely new technique actually—that was being added to the class, and the transmission for it simply couldn't be done at a distance. To receive that new technique, students did need to take a few more days of class. All other class upgrades have been given to students automatically.

8. Do I need to wait for some time between classes to let my system integrate? The transmissions are completely integrated during the time spent in the classes. For some people, though, there is more time that is needed for their energy systems and consciousness to finish processing all the movement that happened in class. Typically this only takes a few days. If in doubt, you can query the teacher of the class in question.

9. If I want to practice VortexHealing, do I need to pay any organizational fees or continue to take VortexHealing classes? Many organizations have these kinds of requirements. VortexHealing does not. We have no organizational fees and no continuing education classes are required to be able to practice VortexHealing or advertise the practice of it.

10. When I channel VortexHealing, do I need to protect myself from picking up my client's 'stuff'? No, you don't need to protect yourself, because you can't really pick up other people's stuff. I am aware that many people believe that you can pick up the stuff that clients release in sessions, but what is really happening is that the channeler is reacting to the receiver's stuff, even if they aren't conscious of doing so. They have their own emotional reactions and then blame it on the client. In addition, when we react to something, we hold it in our peripheral energetic field to keep it away from us. Yet our holding it there also prevents it from moving away from us. A psychic may see the client's emotional charge in the healer's field and tell the healer that they picked up their client's stuff. But it is only there because the healer has reacted to it and is holding it there. The moment the healer lets it go or comes out of their reaction, it moves on and is gone. If you ask enough healers about their experience, you'll find that those who claim they are picking up their clients' stuff will tend to be very choosy about what they pick up. Some will only pick up sadness, some will only pick up anger, and so on. That alone tells you that whatever is going on is more about the healer than what the client is releasing. With VortexHealing, though, the energetic field that is created from bringing through divine energy and consciousness tends to prevent this unconscious process from unfolding. So if a VortexHealer finds, in spite of this, that they are reacting to a particular client, they are taught to own that as their own emotional process and to transform it within their own consciousness.

11. What is VortexHealing's view of traditional Western medicine? We see all forms of medicine as having a role to play in treating someone holistically. Although Western medicine is more focused on the symptoms of disease than the deeper causes, often those symptoms need medical intervention. Although even doctors acknowledge that allopathic drugs are very much over-prescribed, if I were to be in a bad car crash, I would not want to be taken to my local healer; I'd want to go to the nearest hospital. In one VortexHealing class, a student developed a bad strep infection in her hand. It had spread enough that, to my perception, she was really in danger. I sent her to the emergency room.

The strength of Western medicine is its ability to save lives in critical care situations and what it can accomplish with surgery. The strength of holistic healing is being able to get to the true causes of a condition and prevent it from getting to a critical stage.

The VortexHealing view is that traditional Western medicine and alternative healing should be working together, combining their strengths. A truly holistic medicine focuses on both causes and effects, and uses whatever healing modalities will help any given individual patient.

12. Do I need to memorize a lot of material about the energy system to practice VortexHealing? No, you do not. In every class, there are handouts given out that contain step-by-step instructions for a typical session. Yet even this is just a guideline. You can do very deep and powerful sessions just by channeling your highest level of VortexHealing with the simple intention of healing and harmonizing the receiver.

13. Do I need to have any previous training in healing or in the body's energy system to take the Basic/Foundational class? No previous training is required, and any needed information is covered in class.

14. Since Merlin is an expression of Divinity, can't anyone work with Merlin without taking a VortexHealing class? Yes. Merlin is an expression of Divinity and so is available to all. What VortexHealing does, by divine intention, is focus this expression of Divinity so it can be used for healing in a way that people wouldn't be able to create on their own, just by meditating on Merlin. As mentioned earlier, in ancient times Merlin manifested a huge 'divine package' of his energy and consciousness on Earth, with the intention for that to be the foundation of the Merlin lineage here. That package, which focuses Merlin's energy and consciousness for use in VortexHealing, is not available to all. That was a gift specific for the Merlin lineage.

Glossary

Ancestral/Genetic Personality: the aspect of our personality that is inherited from our ancestors, carried in our DNA, in contrast to the aspect of our personality that we have carried over from past lives.

Avatar: an expression of Divinity that can be interacted with as if it were a being, which can also incarnate into a human body.

Awakening: the shift in awareness that happens when the I-sense in the heart permanently disappears, synonymous with the loss of the Core Veil.

Black Hole: a very dense and dark spot in our energy field created when a fear of annihilation or unbearable emotional pain becomes focused and contracted enough to create something that looks like a 'black hole'.

Blueprints: energetic/consciousness structures created by Divinity for how something should grow or unfold in our bodies or our lives, that is manifested into our energy fields and consciousness at higher dimensional levels.

Breaking a TimeLine: happens when the time-continuity of a body, or an area of it, is broken for some moments, making it oscillate in and out of time, enabling Divinity to quickly drain that area of conditioning or even change the course of a person's life.

Core Veil: the construct in our consciousness, sitting in our hearts, that holds our core sense of 'I'.

Divine Web: manifests the vital web and thus creation, continuously feeding it energy and divine intention, maintaining creation and directing its evolution.

Embodiment: the process of learning to live from one's awakening.

Energy Bodies: occupy the same space as our physical bodies but are made up of different densities of 'subtle tissue', with each energy body having its own role and function within our overall energy system.

Energy System: our complete system of energy bodies and energy pathways, including our incarnational body and its energy pathways, all of which forms the basis of our physicality.

Fixations: an emotional and/or energetic structure that can get created when we react to traumatic events, that manifests in consciousness or within the body, with some able to be carried from life to life.

Grounding Cord: an energetic cord that is created from the earth to every human being while they are in the womb that becomes part of their energy system, supporting it and strengthening it, and that helps the person to 'ground' and feel connected to the earth.

Incarnational Personality: the aspect of our personality that we have carried over from past lives, in contrast to the aspect of our personality that is inherited from our ancestors, carried in our DNA.

Intelligence Field: a massive field of intelligence that pervades creation and that has a local expression, a Localized Intelligence Field, for each lifeform.

Karma Knots: the focal points of the incarnational issues and identities, carried by the incarnational self from life to life, which are held in the spine, in the karmic body, when incarnated in a human body.

Karmic Webbing: the incarnational being 'grows' this out of its karma knots as a vehicle for expressing its consciousness and issues into the various energetic levels new form.

Magical Structures: created when Vortex energy has been made dense enough to express as golden-white threads that are full of divine intention, which have a multitude of different uses, both for healing and for restructuring the flow of consciousness in a living space.

Mehindra: the name of the avataric Source of this VortexHealing lineage, while he was incarnated into a human body 5600 years ago.

Merlin: the name of the divine, avataric expression that manifested the VortexHealing lineage.

Merlin's Global Healing Grid: a healing tool from the Magical Structures class that is designed to be used for situations, whether personal or global.

Merlin's Healing Essence: the VortexHealing tool given in the Basic/Foundational class that brings in Merlin's divine consciousness.

Navel Hookup: a way of deepening the energetic connection already present between the channeler and receiver for the duration of a healing.

Running Divine Lines: the VortexHealing tool given in the Basic/Foundational class that gets Merlin to bridge extra divine energy from the divine web into the receiver's vital web, energizing whatever area is being focused on in a healing.

Spot of Non-Existence: created from a 'black hole' (see above), when there is also a deep enough craving for non-existence, which makes the contraction within the black hole become even more intense, damaging the vital webbing there.

Universal Self: the foundation of the personal sense of self, which sits in all of creation.

Vital Energy: the basic energy of life, of livingness, of *I am,* carried in the vital web that is creation.

Vital Web: the manifested energetic structure of creation, which is created and maintained by the divine web.

Vortex Energies: the 49 divine healing energies that can be accessed with the Vortex Wheel, given in the Basic/Foundational class.

Vortex Wheel: the fundamental transmission given in the Basic/ Foundational class, which is the vehicle for the 49 Vortex energies, for Merlin's Healing Essence, and for accessing Merlin for Running Divine Lines.

About the Author

Ric Weinman is the founder of VortexHealing, which he re-discovered in a profound 'vision', November 26, 1994.

Ric grew up in Queens, New York. He went to Columbia University as an engineering student, and in his sophomore year he transferred into its liberal arts college, majoring in English and getting his BA in 1971. In his senior year, he experienced a deep emotional trauma, and when he graduated, he left the country to backpack around Europe and 'find himself'. While traveling, he barely ate and got very far 'out of body', trying to escape his trauma. Yet in his 'out there' and starved state, although he lost a lot of his body mass, his nervous system transformed into a different state and he rediscovered his spiritual connection. As he began the slow journey back into his body, he took this new inner connection with him.

Ric lived 'at the edge' for many years, working odd jobs and day jobs, still barely eating, traveling a lot, but living mostly in Tucson, Arizona. During that time he did a lot of meditation and writing. Some of his short stories were published, with one ending up in a college-level creative writing textbook. He also published two books (*Your Hands Can Heal*, printed in seven languages, and *Breaking the Illusion*). It was in Tucson that his psychic abilities started to activate, and he began to practice healing. He studied Jin Shin Jyutsu®, craniosacral therapy, and practiced his own methods of working with energy, consciousness, and fascia. At one point he began to teach his own healing workshops, which became the basis of his first book, *Your Hands Can Heal*. At that time, he also started to connect inside to various expressions of Divinity. These connections became his main lifeline.

Ric took a short detour into a Masters program in Computer Science at the University of Arizona, attempting to move into a more secure, mainstream existence, but his heart wasn't in it, so he left computer science and returned to his healing work.

Then, in November 1994, his path took a radical turn when, in a profound vision, he found himself standing in a huge interdimensional vortex, and the divine presence within that vortex re-activated his past-life connections to VortexHealing and the Merlin Lineage. People quickly noticed how powerful this healing art was, and they asked him to teach it. In September 1995, he taught the first VortexHealing® Basic/Foundational training, in Tucson.

Almost seven years later, meditating in a hotel room in Colorado, on vacation with his wife and young son, his core sense of 'I' suddenly disappeared. He had been moved into spiritual awakening by the divine Source of his lineage. This began a new phase for both his personal life and for VortexHealing. As his own awakening deepened, he realized he was being shown an awakening map that could be used to take VortexHealing students, step by step, through the same stages that he was being guided through. When the map seemed complete, he wrote *Awakening Through the Veils: A Seeker's Guide,* to share the map with the general spiritual world, along with guidelines for making its journey.

At the time of this writing, Ric lives with his wife and son in Massachusetts.

"VortexHealing made my life smoother. I am no longer an anxious person and a control freak. My family keeps telling me how hard it was to be with me when I was stressed. I am a much happier person now. I am relaxed and I have learned to enjoy every moment."

Mir K., healer. Argentina

"With VortexHealing, my entire physical, mental, psychological, and spiritual systems have been transformed. It has become a path of awakening that calls me every day, and sometimes several times a day, to 'come home'."

Ariane G., Ed.D., creative career coach and writer. USA

"When I started with VortexHealing I wanted to use it as a healing art for my psychotherapy and coaching clients. I ended up going through a huge development within myself. VortexHealing put me, with both feet on the ground, in my body and in my essence. There is more light, space, and freedom in my life, and my understanding and perception are much clearer. I am very grateful for VortexHealing in my life."

Micheline B., psychotherapist, life coach, and healing practitioner. Netherlands

"I didn't believe stories about spirituality, healing and awakening until I experienced VortexHealing. What a blessing to find out that light, peace and inner space was a real option, also for me, even in the worst period of my life."

Jolien S., healer, garden designer, photographer, and politician. Netherlands

"VortexHealing impacted my life as nothing before I had studied or practiced. For the first time, I found deep freedom within myself, and a lot of health and energy. Practicing VortexHealing taught me to surrender deep in life. The result is joy, love and abundance. It's a grace for me to share this with my clients in a full-time VortexHealing practice."

Kristina M., psychologist, energy healing practitioner, and musician. Germany

"VortexHealing has changed my life to love, grace, joy and inner power. It's a permanent process like coming home. It is magical, surprising, fulfilling, and joyful. I'm deeply grateful. I'm in constant touch with the Divine - I had never experienced this before in such an intense way. There's a deep connection to myself, to other people, and to the whole universe. VortexHealing is the best thing that has happened to me in this life."

Regina O., psychotherapist. Germany

www.ingramcontent.com/pod-product-compliance
Lightning Source LLC
Chambersburg PA
CBHW020521290526
45786CB00002B/703